Macrobiotics:
An
Invitation
To Health
And Happiness

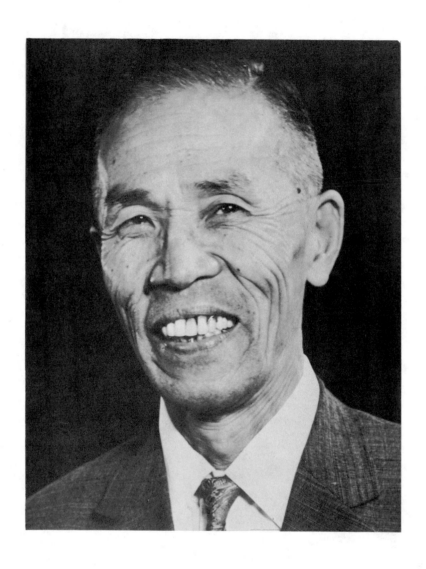

George   Ohsawa

Macrobiotics: An Invitation To Health And Happiness

by George Ohsawa

Herman Aihara, Editor

Photograph by Jacques de Langre

GEORGE OHSAWA MACROBIOTIC FOUNDATION INC.: PUBLISHERS

Published by the George Ohsawa
Macrobiotic Foundation
1544 Oak Street
Oroville, California
95965

First Printing June 1971
Second Printing September 1971
Third Printing 1976
Fourth Printing 1976
Fifth Printing September 1978

Printed in the U.S.A.
ISBN 09-18860-01-4

CONTENTS

正食は世上の一道なり
始めあるそノにオワリあり、
表するそノたウラあり
表大なれバウラも亦大なり
　　　　如一

Note on the Illustrations

PREFACE

Oriental science and philosophy are practical and useful. The latter is Macrobiotics, which I am going to introduce to you in this book. The former is physiognomy of which I will teach you so that you can grasp what Oriental science is. Oriental science includes medicine based on the observation of phenomena. Deduction of the theory, however, is based on a principle of life or the Order of the Universe: Yin and Yang. By using the Yin-Yang principle, each science or philosophy can relate to practical daily life, and will not lose their way into analytical sectionalism and academic knowledge.

Western science has also tried to start establishing happiness in Man. Due to the lack of the fundamental life principle, however, it has reached confusion in trying to solve many problems - cancer, heart diseases, mental diseases, diabetes, drug use, abortion, birth control, allergy, crime, social disorders, pollution, over-population, poverty, etc.

Whatever problems we want to solve, we should start with ourselves. This is the Oriental approach. A happy society must be built on happy individuals. Everyone's happiness depends on his health. One's health is his physical constitution and condition which are manifested in his face, eyes, nose, ears, hair, etc.

Oriental physiognomy is based on biology, physiology, and embryology. It is useful and amazing. It tells one's fate by his face and bone structure. Macrobiotics teaches the mechanism of such physical formations. Therefore, one can create physical happiness as well as change poor health to good.

Man is a free animal who can change his fate. Macrobiotics is a teaching of the way of this change. He who doesn't know how to change must remain a slave to money, to a job; a man who lives life monotonously and mechanically, and depends solely on fame and status. If you want to be free from such dependency, you must be healthy first. This book is for people whose aim is health and happiness, *by* and *for* himself.

For such people, the Oriental physiognomy is useful. Here is its "short-cut" secret:

1. Ears

One whose ear lobe is large will have a happier life. One whose ear lobe is clear cut from his face will have good luck, longevity, and security in life. One who doesn't have an ear lobe will be unhappy. Happiness is one who has ears which are flat against the side of his face so that they can rarely be seen from the front. Unhappiness is one whose ears are wide like a rabbit.

2. Eyes

A man becomes happier when he has small and thin eyes (like a slit). A woman becomes happier when she has small but round eyes and brightly opened. Extruding eyes are a symptom of a weak heart. Such eyes are a sign of irregular menstruation in women. They foretell a difficult life for either man or woman.

3. Sanpaku Eyes

Observation of the eye is the first step of Oriental physiognomy.

a. This eye is the sign of great vitality of the rising sun. He who has this eye doesn't know fear or insecurity. All babies are like this.

b. This is a normal eye. He who has this eye can be healthy and happy.

c. This is the beginning of Sanpaku because white starts to appear between the lower side of the iris and the lower lid. One who has this eye starts to show sluggishness.

d. Complete Sanpaku. One who has this eye is suspicious, fearful, insecure, quick to misunderstand, and passive. His heart, sexual organs, liver, kidney, and lungs are very sick. He cannot keep promises, wastes time, has a bad memory, is prone to accidents and a miserable death. Lincoln, J. F. Kennedy, Hitler, Lenin, Stalin, Tyrone Power, Marilyn Monroe were all Sanpaku. Most political leaders have such eyes. This is the main cause of the world crises and struggles that exist today. The persons on wanted posters in post offices in the United States have such Sanpaku eyes. Most of the criminals, thieves, suicides, and other persons wanted by the F.B.I. are Sanpaku.

e. When one dies the black part goes way up. This is the sign of death.

If a taxi driver is Sanpaku, it is better to avoid a ride in his car. Watch your opponent with whom you discuss or negotiate because he is tricky. The final winner is always he who is not Sanpaku.

One who has Sanpaku eyes must cure it as soon as possible. Watch your better half's eyes. If he or she is Sanpaku, you must change it. Otherwise, your marriage will be unhappy.

Man's Sanpaku - Impotence

Woman's Sanpaku - Irregularity in ovaries, irregularity of menstruation, malformation of the womb, dislike of sex, inability to conceive.

4. Shape of the Face

A man's face should have an oval shape, as do grains. A square shape is the face of carnivorous animals - for instance, a tiger or cat. One who has a △ shaped face is aggressive, active, joyous, but sometimes violent. It is good for men but not for women because it will lead her to separation or divorce.

One who has a ▽ shaped face is passive, shy, lacking in courage and decision. He is often exclusive and unhappy. A man's face is normally shorter than a woman's. A woman's face is normally longer than a man's.

5. Hair

One who has red hair is tempermental. Grey hair is the result of too much animal foods. He has a tendency to have a brain hemorrage, heart attack, rheumatism, and arthritis. Fallen hair is a sign of excess Vitamin C and indicates weak sex power.

6. Baldness

Baldness of the forehead is caused by an excess of Vitamin C and indicates impotency or a weak heart. Baldness on the top of the head is caused by excess animal protein and signifies short temper, roughness, and an inclination toward too much sexual activity.

7. Skin

Skin that is smooth, has a good complexion and is resistable to any injury is a sign of good health. Dirty skin (acne, rash-prone, rough, or that which has any disease) is mostly caused by excess sugar. Pale skin is caused by excess fruit.

8. Body Hair

A woman who grows hair below the nose, and is hairy on either the arms or legs is diseased in the ovaries or womb. She may have trouble in menstruation and lack ovary hormones. She may sometimes produce male hormones. She is a male-female who will not have a lasting marriage; she will be divorced soon. There is a female-male too, who is not able to satisfy his mate. Therefore, he will not have a happy life.

MACROBIOTICS:
AN INVITATION TO HEALTH AND HAPPINESS

INTRODUCTION

It seems to me that man's ultimate desire is happiness. I rarely find a person, however, whose life is really happy. Many live in complaint, discontent, fear, and despair. Even a happy person rarely can continue to be happy more than a year or two, without having a car accident, a divorce, a separation, heart attack, or cancer. If he is happy for about ten years, he must be kept in a museum because such a person has become extinct in our society.

Were we born in this world to suffer and to spend miserable, unhappy lives for seventy or eighty years? How miserable we are, if we spend even a short time of life in fear and insecurity, agony and sadness!

Here I introduce to you a simple and practical diet which will lead you to a joyous, happy, and wonderful life. This diet was a basic principle of major Oriental religions until the intellectuality of Western man discarded such practical teaching and the development of science and technology overshadowed its usefulness.

My aim in writing this small booklet is to introduce you to the way of eating and selection of foods which will eventually lead you to true, eternal happiness.

I. What is Happiness

First of all we need to learn only one thing - nothing else: happiness. Everyone is seeking happiness. What is the definition of happiness?

There are various Occidental definitions of happiness (from the Syntopicon). According to Kant, "The principle of private happiness is the direct opposite of the principle of morality." He understood happiness to consist in "the satisfaction of all our desires." Hence, there is no universal

1

solution to the problem of how to be happy.

According to Locke, "Though all men's desires tend to happiness, yet they are not moved by the same object. Men may choose different things, and yet all choose right." The ancient philosophers with whom Locke disagrees insist that a science of ethics depends on a first principle which is self-evident in the same way to all men. Happiness is not that principle if the content of happiness is what each man thinks it to be; for no universally applicable definition of happiness can be given. With their conception of what constitutes happiness, one man may be as right as another. Then the fact that all men agree upon giving the name "happiness" to what they ultimately want amounts to no more than a nominal agreement. Such nominal agreement, in the opinion of Aristotle and Aquinas, does not suffice to establish a science of ethics, with rules for the pursuit of happiness which shall apply universally to all men. The most obvious mark of the happy man according to Aristotle is that he wants nothing, or he has everything. The happy life leaves nothing to be desired. Aquinas defined happiness the same as Aristotle.

According to Plotinus, happiness is one with justice because justice, or virtue in general, is "the health and beauty and well-being of the soul." This association of happiness with health - the one, a harmony in the soul as the other, a harmony in the body - appears also in Freud's consideration of human well-being. For Freud, the ideal of health - not merely bodily health, but the health of the whole man - seems to identify happiness with peace of mind. "Anyone who is born with an especially unfavorable instinctual constitution," he writes, "and whose libido-components do not go through the transformation and modification necessary for successful achievement in later life, will find it hard to obtain happiness." Freud is right to think that achievement of happiness depends on the physical condition. However, he doesn't define this happiness.

Mill considered the achievement of happiness from the point of economics and politics. Since happiness of man is limited by political states and economical conditions, Mill's view is that happiness is an illusory goal. Such a conclusion

2

on happiness brings up the theological consideration of happiness. According to theologians, perfect happiness belongs to the eternal life of the immortal soul which is at rest in the vision of God and unites the infinite good.

According to Occidental definitions, therefore, happiness is very unhappy. They are all too conceptual, philosophical, or stoic. There are so many different answers and in the end, they say that true peace of soul can be found only by rare individuals and that happiness is an illusory goal. It seems to me that no one clearly defines what happiness is. It is obvious why so much tragedy has been produced in the Western world. Do you agree with the conceptions of the West or the "Light from the East"?

There were hundreds of great philosophers in China some thousands of years ago. They collaborated to coin the Chinese definition of happiness:

1. To live in interesting, amusing, joyful longevity without knowing old age.

2. Not to be worried about money.

3. To have calmness, tranquility of mind. Not to get angry or emotionally upset by any accidents, trage-dies, or difficulties. Lack of such calmness may cause premature death.

4. To have much gratitude and to love to put everything in order. To be a good organizer and generous giver.

5. Not to be the first, who will later be the last. (It is said in the Bible, "The first will become the last and the last will become the first. But be the last who will be the first in the end and forever.") To have humility, to be a very modest and moderate person.

What do you think of this Chinese definition of happiness? For me, this is too complicated, too scholarly, too intellect-ual, too philosophical and metaphysical.

The Indian people coined another definition of happiness that is "Maka Hannya Haramitta Sutra" (or "Maka Prajuna

3

Haramitta Shingyo", see *The Supreme Judgment Taught by Buddha* published by GOMF). It consists of only 262 words. It is very difficult to understand this Sutra. This is the essence of Buddha's teaching. According to Buddha, we have eight types of sufferings:

A. Biological and Physiological sufferings.
  1. Pain and suffering from living.
  2. Sickness.
  3. Suffering and old age.
  4. Pain and suffering of death.

B. Psychological sufferings.
  1. Suffering from the separation from one's loved one sooner or later.
  2. Suffering from hatred.
  3. Desires that attract all temptations in this world. (Man's temptations such as seeking beautiful women, delicious foods, delicious drink, comfortable house and luxurious car, etc. cause anxiety, worry and unsatisfied agony in him.)
  4. Suffering from incapacity and frustration of not getting what one wants.

To abolish all these eight sufferings of man, Buddha invented a new teaching called "Buddhism" which teaches us to attain happiness through eight righteous ways. In Buddhism, happiness is defined as "Satori" or "Nirvana".

My own definition of happiness is to do anything one wants and enjoy it day and night up to the end of his life, realizing all his dreams and being loved by all during life and even after death. Such life is happiness itself.

If you agree I will give you a key to enter such a happy land. It seems impossible to have such a life. Mr. Eastman of Kodak committed suicide. Even Thomas Edison was very sad toward the end of his life. He was desperate. He said after 80 years, "I devoted all my life inventing 6,000 inventions. All were made to promote happiness for people, but now I see the world is no happier than it was 80 years ago." Gandhi fought all his life without weapons against the British Empire, and he conquered. He is like a God in India and the world. But even he died desperately. He realized the liberation of all Indians, but India was divided and separated. He wished to be killed as soon as possible. There are many examples like this unhappiness. But I guarantee you your happiness. Its way is Macrobiotics. In America, there are hundreds of people who have completely renewed their life and begun a new one.

II. Judgment and Health

THE SEVEN STAGES (or LEVELS) of JUDGMENT

STAGE	UNDERSTANDING	LOVE
7) Supreme	Enlightenment Self-realization Do (Aiki-do, etc.) Satori, Cosmic Consciousness	All-embracing (no preferences; finds nothing at all intolerable)
6) Idealogical	Philosophy, religion, dialectics	Spiritual
5) Social	Ethics, Morality, Economics	Social
4) Intellectual	Science, some of the arts	Scientific (of know-ledge, research)
3) Sentimental	Literature, theatre, most arts	Emotional, Psychological
2) Sensorial	Dance, gymnastics, Conditioned reflex	Physiological, physical, erotic sensual, sensory
1) Mechanical	Instinctive, unconscious reflex; no understanding	Instinctual (no discretion; only blind appetite)

(In Japanese, there is at least one word for each of the seven stages of Love described above.)

Note:
1. He who saves money or property for himself or children is using "minus" 7th level of judgment.
2. He who hates or betrays is on the minus 3rd level of judgment.
3. He who has special likings (food, drink, etc.) is using the 2nd level of judgment.
4. He who lives on the knowledge of science and religion is on the 2nd level of judgment. However, he who studies

PROFESSION	WAY OF EATING
Happy man who amuses himself throughout his life, realizing all his dreams	Anything he wants with great joy and gratitude
Originator of ideas, thinker, writer, lecturer	According to a dietetic or religious principle
Organizer	Conformist
Seller of knowledge and techniques	According to the currently fashionable nutritional theory
Seller of emotions	Gourmet (connoisseur)
Seller of pleasure; prostitute, actor, merchant, advertising man	Gourmand (greedy)
Seller of his life; Working slave; salary earner	Guided by hunger and thirst alone

such knowledge for intellectual growth is on the 4th level of judgment.

5. He who dislikes something or someone and is always difficult and complaining is lower than the 6th level.
6. He who welcomes difficulties and challenges is able to reach Supreme Judgment.
7. He whose aim in life is to reach Satori or Highest Health is a candidate for the 7th level of judgment.

In order to attain happiness, one must reveal highest judgment and health. The way which leads one to this is Macrobiotics. This is a way of living by following instruction derived from the Order of the Universe or the Principle of Unification.

The Macrobiotic diet improves health and clear thinking. Therefore, it improves efficiency of study or work. He who observes the Macrobiotic diet has no fatigue and therefore can work twice as effectively and accomplish twice as much as other people. Everyone likes him because he can maintain a good disposition. With Macrobiotics, athletic men can improve their skill and record in swimming, marathons, baseball, etc.; artists can show rapid progress in painting, music, dancing, martial arts, etc. Men who have dark, gloomy faces will show brightness and intelligence. Women become younger, more beautiful, and grow abundant hair. They will give birth to as many children as they wish. They can even select the sex of the baby who will be born.

III. Seven Conditions of Health (Self-diagnosis of Health)

Before observing my dietetic directions, it would be wise for you to evaluate the state of your health in accordance with the seven conditions that follow. The first three conditions are physiological: if you satisfy them all, you score fifteen points or five points for each. The fourth, fifth, and sixth, psychological in nature, are valued at ten points each. The seventh and most important condition of all is worth fifty-five points. In all, there are a total of one hundred points. Be sure to do this self-consultation before you try the Macrobiotic diet and again one month or two months later.

1. No Fatigue: 5 points
You should not feel fatigued. If you catch cold, your organism has been tired for many years. Even one cold in ten years is a bad sign for there is no bird or insect that ever catches colds, even in cold countries and cold weather. Fatigue manifests itself in mentality too. If you are prone to saying, "It is too difficult, It is impossible, or I am not prepared for such a thing," you reveal your tiredness.

8

If you are really healthy, you can overpower and chase away difficulties one after the other, as a dog chases a rabbit. If you tend to avoid difficulties, however, then you are a defeatest.

We must be adventurers in life since tomorrow is an unknown world. The bigger the difficulty, the bigger the pleasure. This attitude is the sign of freedom from fatigue.

Fatigue is the real foundation of all diseases. You can cure it without any medicine if you understand and practice the Macrobiotic way to longevity and rejuventation.

2. Good Appetite: 5 points

If you cannot take any kind of simple food with the deepest gratitude to the Creator, God, with joy and pleasure, it indicates that you are lacking appetite. If you can find simple brown rice or whole bread very appetizing then you have a good appetite and a healthy stomach. Good appetite is health itself.

Sexual appetite and joyful satisfaction are an essential condition of happiness. If a man or woman has no sexual appetite and pleasure, it means he or she is violating the natural order of man which is a specific manifestation of the Order of the Universe - Yin and Yang. Violation of man's order (original writing reads "violation of the Order of the Universe") through ignorance can only lead to sickness and insanity. Those who are impotent hate sexuality. All those who are vexed and angry, inside or out, can never enter the Kingdom of Heaven.

3. Deep and Good Sleep: 5 points

If you speak or have dreams and nightmares in your sleep, your sleep is not deep and good. If you are entirely satisfied with four to six hours of sleep then your sleep is healthy. If you cannot get profound sleep within three or four minutes after putting your head on the pillow, under any circumstances, at any time, it shows that your mind is not free from fear. If you cannot get up at the time you wish (fixed in your mind before going to bed), it indicates that your sleep was imperfect.

4. Good Memory: 10 points

If you do not forget anything that you see or hear, it is a sign of good health. With Macrobiotic dialectical directions, you can re-establish and strengthen your memory infinitely. Memory is the most important factor of our life as it is the basic foundation of our Judgment. The good Yogi, or the Buddhist or Christian saint always has infinite memory. They can even visualize their anterior life. You can see this in a diabetic patient who has lost his memory on account of his disease. By observing Macrobiotic instructions the diabetic patient will regain his lost memory very rapidly. This is true not only of the diabetic patient; even an idiot, imbecile or neurasthenic can regain his original memory. Macrobiotic students easily achieve good grades because of good memory. We have many examples of this. Through memory, we can gain good judgment and then happiness. Good memory is the foundation of happiness.

5. Good Humor (freedom from anger): 10 points

A man of good health should be cheerful and pleasant under any circumstances. One should be without fear and suffering. Such a man will be more happy, brave and enthusiastic even with growing and accumulating difficulties and enemies. Your appearance, your voice, your behavior, and even your criticism should display deep gratitude and thankfulness to all those who are in your presence. All your words should be an expression of your deep gratitude and joy, as the poems of Tagore. We should be happy and in good humor like a boy with a magnificent present before him. If we are not, this shows that we lack good health. The healthy person never gets angry!

If you have any insignificant complaint of a mental, physiological or social nature or if you don't have many intimate and loyal friends, it would be wise to observe my directions and eat a small portion of Kombu or Wakame (without cooking) to neutralize the acidity of your body. You can see the truth of this statement by experimenting on one of your children. Stop giving sugar, honey, ice cream, chocolate, etc., which acidify his blood. A very Yin child will turn into a very Yang and joyful child in a week or two.

We rarely meet with men of agreeable temperament. The majority of men and women are sick, but they are not to be blamed because they don't know how to attain good humor. They don't know what they should eat and drink, and how.

You can give good humor, a smile, an agreeable voice and the simple words "thank you" infinitely. You lose nothing at all, because you have received life itself and everything in this Universe without pay. You are the unique son or daughter of the Infinite Universe. If you know this, you will be loved by all.

If you are cheerful and loved by all, always and everywhere, giving more and more to others and especially the biggest and best thing in this world, you will be happiest. There will be one among millions who will express the greatest joy. You can achieve this if you observe my directions. My Macrobiotic medicine is in reality a kind of Alladin's lamp or flying carpet. To realize this joyful good temper, you must first of all re-establish your health.

6. Smartness in Thinking and Doing: 10 points

A man who is in good health should have the faculty of correct thinking, judgment, and doing with promptness and smartness. Promptness is the expression of Freedom. Those who are prompt, speedy and precise, and those who are ready to answer to any challenge, accident or necessity are in good health.

They distinguish themselves by their ability to establish order everywhere in the kingdom of animals and vegetables is an expression of the order of the plant or animal.

Man's health and happiness are expressions of the order of man which is part of the Order of the Universe. (The Order of the Universe expresses itself as health and sickness in man.) Physical orderliness of man is health. Mental orderliness in man is happiness. To establish this order of man is the aim of the Macrobiotic diet. You can cure not only physical disease, but also mental or moral diseases by observing these simple Macrobiotic directions, which are the essence of wisdom five thousand years old. Do you have a more modern method? I don't know of one more direct and simple than ours. If I am wrong in my judgment, please tell me. If so, I am ready to follow you, and give up the biological, physiological, and cosmological way of "health to peace" that I have followed joyfully for 48 years (since 1912).

7. Honesty: 55 points

One who never tells a lie, keeps promises and appointments, is never suspicious, and who is eager to follow justice is honest. He who devotes his whole life to reveal truth - that which does not change - and who teaches others by his deeds that liers, double talkers, doubtful and suspicious persons inevitably end up very unhappy, is honest.

He who lives a life in search of eternal truth, overcoming all superstition and hypotehtical thinking, and tries to reveal the beautiful and eternal truth in this relative and ephemeral world, is honest. Such an honest man is healthy. Who thinks himself to be honest has 55 points by this test alone.

How much is your score in the self-examination of health - 40 points, 20 points, or zero? Don't worry. You can improve your health by observing the Macrobiotic diet. In fact, one who gives himself a low score is an honest person. Therefore, his health amounts to at least 55 points. He who gives himself more than 60 points does not need to read my book further. Good bye.

IV. Food for Health and Happiness

The way to realize the seven conditions of health and happiness described in the previous chapter is Macrobiotics, a diet based on a practical life principle. Macrobiotics is a modernization of ancient Sen-Do, a Way of Longevity. It is a gyo, which is one of the eight right ways to reach Satori.

Modern medicine has progressed more in the past one hundred years than in the two thousand years following its introduction by Hippocrates. It has conquered the world.

Contrary to its progress, however, the health of man has never improved. The number of incurable diseases and chronically ill patients has increased. Many of the leaders of the cancer institutes and hospitals in Japan have died from cancer. Mental patients amount to almost half of the sick in America.

There are many diets for health in America:

1. The nutritional theory which was started by Voit, a German physiologist, about 90 years ago, is based on the caloric theory. The nutritionist labeled the basic nutritions needed by man as protein carbohydrates and fat. To this list, vitamins, enzymes, and minerals have recently been added.

2. Health food diets stress the importance of vitamins and they recommend vitamin intake through food supplements. From the Macrobiotic point of view, however, since vitamin supplements are extracts or synthetic chemicals, they are not even partial foods or not foods at all.

3. People who observe vegetarian, fruitarian, and raw food diets claim that vegetables should not be cooked because heat destroys the value of foods by destroying the vitamins and enzymes. Many health food followers are against the Macrobiotic diet from this point of view. They overlook three things: a. The fact is that they are reacting to the previous heavy meat-eating diet. They have previously eaten so much meat and have become so yang that they are attracted to Yin - raw vegetables and fruit. b. It is also true that the vitamins and enzymes in raw foods are destroyed in our digestive process. Therefore, this diet doesn't have sound reasoning. c. The Macrobiotic diet never excludes raw foods. There are many recipes for salads which can be eaten according to climate, season, and other food combinations.

4. High protein diets are symptomatic and are derived from the osmotic pressure theory and may be valid in certain cases for a limited period.

5. The mucusless diet is probably good for those who are meat-eaters or have been heavy meat-eaters in the past. Although the mucusless diet has good reasoning and results for certain people, it tends to be symptomatic.

6. Juice is an extraction from food, and therefore is not whole. The juice diet is a degenerative one; it will degenerate the intestinal functions.

7. The salt-free diet is also a reaction to a previous diet. It is good for the person who is too yang and has been eating an excess of meat. Except for a few very yang persons, grain-eaters and vegetarians need a proper amount of salt in their diet.

If you're not satisfied with any of these diets, or if you cannot improve your health by any other methods, try the Macrobiotic diet for only a few days. If it is agreeable with you, try another three months. If you feel better, then try one year. The Macrobiotic diet is not dangerous if not observed too rigidly. It is inexpensive and can eliminate all medical expenses. It is a diet of eating only the necessary foods for man.

What are the necessary foods for man? Good air, water, and sunshine are necessary for man to sustain life. Lacking one of them will lead to destruction of the human being. Therefore, these are the most important foods. Other foods which are necessary to man, such as grains, vegetables, beans, seaweeds, and fishes are products or transformations of these 3 basic foods.

The right foods for man are those which are traditionally eaten, locally grown, and seasonal in that particular location. In other words, the right foods for man agree with the ecological law. Man, like any other living thing, is a product of nature, a biological creature. Therefore, he must observe biological and ecological laws, which tell us that soil produces vegetables and grasses, which in turn sustain the life of animals. Therefore, as ancient Chinese believed: the soil and our body are inseparably related. The first Macrobiotic principle, that our food must be locally grown and in season, is drawn from this relationship. In most cases, the traditional foods are good in a particular locality because they have been tested by thousands of people since ancient times (see "8 Principles of Macrobiotics", page 60).

The principle food of the Macrobiotic diet is whole grain because it is a combination of seeds and fruits. It is abundant on the earth. It is the most economical and nutritious food. Only a whole grain diet will solve the starvation problem due to over-population, because 4000 lbs. of grain can be produced per acre, while only 200 lbs. of meat can be produced per acre.

Grains include brown rice, wheat, wholewheat flour, millet, buckwheat, buckwheat flour, barley, rye, oats, whole noodles, and corn, all in their natural state.

Secondary foods are locally and seasonally grown vegetables and seaweeds. Seaweeds can be eaten in an area hundreds of miles away from the ocean because the ocean is our internal environment. Therefore, seaweeds can agree with our internal environment even though one lives far away from the water. Also the composition of the ocean is not affected much by the location, seasons, or weather. However, seaweed grown in a cold current is more yang than that grown in a warm current.

The condiments used are as follows:

1. Unrefined salt. It this is not available, add seaweed powder to sea salt at a ratio of about one to one, or add a pinch of moshio (especially processed seaweed powder) to a pint of authentic soy sauce.

2. Oil (sesame oil, corn oil, olive oil, etc.).

3. Miso (traditional).

4. Soy sauce (not chemically made).

5. Kombu soup stock.

6. Dried fish soup stock.

Fish, fowl, shellfish, eggs, and fruits can be used from time to time. However, the Yin-Yang balance of dishes, individual conditions and weather must be considered (see "8 Principles of Macrobiotics"). Dairy products and honey can be used as a pleasure food.

The foods to avoid are products of chemical fertilizer and sprays, synthetic or mass produced foods, products of different localities and seasons, hot-house products, colored, preserved, bleached, artificially sweetened products and those seasoned by chemicals.

In cooking, any style - Chinese, Japanes, French, American, etc. - can be applied in the Macrobiotic diet (see Appendix). Use your creativity and originality. Apply the Yin-Yang principle in your kitchen. Here is endless joy.

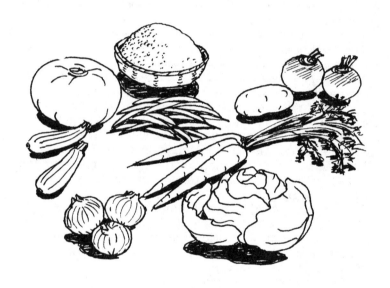

V. How to Eat

Chew well! That is the best policy. He who is sick or who wants to be beautiful and smart must chew well before anything else. Chew each mouthful of food 50 to 100 times. Chewing makes the food delicious. Chewing gives you the real taste of food. By chewing you can distinguish between good food and bad; real food tastes better the more you chew. One person cured himself of cancer in Japan by only chewing well. Chewing well increases not only health but also mental and spiritual clarity. Judgment improves. "Eat your drink, and drink your food."

VI. Macrobiotic External Treatment

1. Ginger fomentation:
Place 4 oz. of raw grated ginger or 1 heaping tsp. of dried powder in a cotton sack. Drop sack into ½ to 1 gallon of water which is just below boiling point. Squeeze a towel in this yellow hot water and make fomentation on any painful part. Cover this with a big bath towel so that it will not cool off easily. If this is too hot for you, first cover your skin with another towel and then apply the hot towel over it. Change the towel 3 or 4 times during 15 minutes. This is effective for painful or swollen parts especially for rheumatism, congestion, convulsions, colitis, kidney troubles, etc. It improves blood circulation.

2. Albi (Sato-imo) plaster:
Albi is an Indian name. It is called Yucca in America, Sato-imo in Japan, and Taro in Africa. Add the same volume of wholewheat flour and 10% raw ginger to grated albi. Stretch this plaster on a sheet of paper or cloth. The plaster must be ½ inch thick. Cover the painful part amply with this plaster. You can cover this plaster with another cloth for several hours. This must be applied after ginger fomentation. Do this 4 or 5 times a day. This application will be made on the inflamed or painful parts. It is effective in curing tuberculosis, appendicitis, rheumatism, arthritis, tumors and excema. It is also effective in curing such diseases as leprosy and cancer.

3. Tofu plaster (Soybean curd):
Squeeze tofu and add 10% wheat flour. Stretch this

directly on any painful part with inflammation. All fever, pain, or inflammation will soon be relieved.

4. Sesame ginger.
Mix one spoonful of sesame oil and another spoonful of ginger juice well. This is very good for headaches, and at the same time stops falling hair and dandruff.

5. Pure sesame oil.
Filter sesame oil with cotton, cheese cloth, or gauze. Apply one drop of this to your eye before sleeping. It is very good for all eye sicknesses.

6. Hip bath #1.
Cook 2 or 3 Hiba (dried leaves of 2 or 3 white Japanese radishes) in 1 gallon of water with a handful of salt. Cover your hip warmly with this hot water. Add more hiba water from time to time to keep the water hot. This is a chlorophyll bath. Have a cup of Soy-Ban (soy sauce in Bancha tea) after taking this bath, 10 to 15 minutes before going to bed. This is very good for all female sexual organ diseases, such as leukorrhea, diseases of the uterus, and of the ovaries.

7. Hip bath #2
Make the above mentioned hip bath without hiba, but with salt.

8. Ginger hip bath.
Grate 1 lb. of ginger. Put it in a sack of cotton. Boil this with 2 gallons of water. This is very good for violent dysentery. If it is not so violent, make half the quantity. Squeeze a towel in it, and apply this hot compress on the abdomen.

9. Salt compress.
Heat 2 or 3 lbs. of salt. Put it in a cotton sack or cloth. Apply this on the painful part of your body.

10. Konnyaku fomentation.
Boil 2 or 3 lbs. of Konnyaku and apply it wrapped with two towels on the painful part.

11. Soybean plaster.
Soak a cup of soybeans in water for one night (5 parts water). Crush this and add a little flour. Apply this on the forehead if you have a fever or on any inflammation. It absorbs fever miraculously.

12. Carp plaster.
Take one lb. of carp. Cut off the head and catch the blood coming out in a cup. Have the patient suffering from acute pneumonia drink this before the blood coagulates. Crush the rest very thoroughly and apply this on the chest. Measure the temperature every 30 minutes. When it has returned to normal (within 5 to 6 hours) take off the plaster. Many people have been cured by this method, after having tried all antibiotic drugs in vain.

13. Chlorophyl plaster.
Crush watercress, spinach or big leaves of any green vegetables in a plaster. Apply this plaster on the forehead to absorb fever.

14. Tea fomentation.
Roast Bancha-twig tea and make tea. Add 5% salt. Make a fomentation with this tea on your eye for 10 to 15 minutes, three times a day. It is good for all eye diseases.

15. Dentie.
Salt the head of a sliced eggplant and dry, and then burn. Use these ashes as tooth paste. Apply this to the painful tooth. The pain will be instantly relieved. If you are suffering from pyorrhea, brush your teeth with Dentie and apply to your gums (outside only) before going to bed every night.

16. Rice plaster.
Crush whole rice (raw) with a little water. Apply this directly to the painful wound.

APPENDIX

by Herman Aihara

A. History of Macrobiotics

Almost all Americans are recent immigrants to America. Therefore, most of their dishes came from Europe. However, immigrants from other continents which had various industrial and commercial developments, brought new styles of cuisine to this country which differ greatly from that of Europe. Today, there is a Chinese restaurant in almost any town in America. The Indian philosophy, Yoga, coined the natural health food concept and made fruitarianism and raw-vegetarianism popular in this country. The recent health food trends make up hundreds of different kinds of diets, one being the mucusless diet. They are all alike in one respect; they are all reactions to each other. When one tires of a diet, he changes to its opposite.

There is an entirely new diet, however, started in this mechanically-minded America. This is the Macrobiotic diet. This diet is so unique that all Americans must be taught how to start. The uniqueness of this diet lies not only in its five-thousand-year history but also in its concepts, selection of foods, and way of cooking.

Thousands of years ago, Oriental wise men realized that the food we eat not only sustains life but also creates health and happiness; they compiled religious or medical laws: Code of Manu in India, Ne-Ching in China, Honso-Komoku (the first medicinal herb book) in China, the Zen diet, etc.

Around the beginning of the century, a Japanese doctor, Sagen Ishizuka, established the theory of nutrition and medicine based on the Oriental diet, applying Western science - chemistry, biology, biochemistry, medicine and physiology. His health diet was so popular, that hundreds of patients gathered every day in front of his home, where he prescribed a diet for the sick. When he died, his funeral procession was followed by a line of people several miles long who wanted to salute him. He was born weak and suffered from diseases. In order to improve his health, he studied thousands of books in the West and East. Through life-long study, he wrote two books - *Chemical Theory of Longevity* and *Biochemical Way to Health and Happiness*. After his death (about 60 years ago), a Macrobiotic association was established by his followers. Due to the lack of a great leader, however, this association started to decline. At that time, George Ohsawa, then 22 years old, having been saved by the diet, took over the association and brought it back again to a successful state. After that, Mr. Ohsawa devoted his entire life to preaching the Oriental philosophy and its application all over the world, until his death at the age of 74. Macrobiotics is now practiced in France, Belgium, England, Germany, Norway, Sweden, Brazil, Argentina, Africa, Viet Nam, and India as well as Japan and the United States.

Ohsawa wrote about 300 books in his lifetime, most of them self-publications. He published a monthly magazine for more than 40 years. More than 30 of his books and 23 magazines are now translated into English, German, French, Swedish, Flemish, Portuguese, Italian, and Viet Namese.

In America, thousands of Macrobiotics live around Boston, New York, Seattle, and the San Francisco Bay area. Thousands of health food stores and natural food stores throughout the nation are selling Macrobiotic foods. Order of the Universe in Boston is publishing two periodicals, *The Order of the Universe* and "East-West Journal". The George Ohsawa Macrobiotic Foundation in San Francisco also publishes two periodicals, "Musubi" and *The Macrobiotic*. There are many Macrobiotic books and pamphlets that are available in many stores. Swan House Publishing Co. plans to publish all of Mr. Ohsawa's books in the near future.

There are lecture meetings in various cities (see "Musubi" for further information). Many chiropractic doctors are suggesting the Macrobiotic diet to their patients and getting good results. Dr. Knut of Kansas City told me that he cured about 20 cancer patients in a few years.

Macrobiotics is becoming a social movement in this

country. Many universities and colleges are serving Macrobiotic meals in their cafeterias. The Macrobiotic diet is not a
fad. It is a way of life, even in this "far-out" country. This
small booklet, I hope, will guide you to the road of health
and happiness.

B. Warning with Respect to Diet #7

In the February 1968 issue of McCall's magazine, an
article entitled "10 Diets to Stay Away From" written by a
Harvard nutritional authority, Dr. F. J. Stare, was published
in *The Macrobiotic Monthly* (Vol. 8, #2 issue). I made
comments about his article in order to clarify some misunderstandings of his, as well as those of many Americans. This
article may suggest some advice for Americans on how to
start Macrobiotics:
    "First, I wish to express my thanks to Dr. Stare. Not only
will his warning about the Macrobiotic diet be beneficial to
the American people but also to the growth and development
of Macrobiotics in this country. The beginner will start
cautiously, and experienced Macrobiotics will be provoked
into deeper thought.
    However, since Dr. Stare, like most Americans, is quite a
stranger to this diet, there are several misunderstandings in
his article. Therefore, I feel obligated to clarify these and in
so doing, give Americans a better understanding of this diet. I
do not blame Dr. Stare for his misunderstanding. I am,
rather, in complete sympathy. It is understandable that the
simplicity of the Macrobiotic diet is difficult to comprehend.
    America is the last continent on which rice was cultivated.
It has been about five thousand years since the wild grass of
India was found. This wild grass was turned into the many
varieties of cultivated rice we have today. From India, where
rice has grown for thousands of years, cultivation spread
eastward through China, Japan, Siam, and many islands of
the Far East. The Arabs brought it to Spain and from Spain it
spread throughout Europe. Although rice was unknown in

North America when the colonists landed, there existed a species quite similar. Actual rice, however, was not grown here until the end of the 17th century. In about 1697, Landgrave Thomas Smith produced the first rice in this country. Today some of the finest rice in the world is grown in the United States. According to the 1964 statistics of the Department of Agriculture, the quantity of rice produced in this country is only two per cent of the world production. Although one half of the human population depends on rice for their principal food, Americans remain strangers to this important grain - economically, socially, biologically, and physiologically.

Americans, as well as Europeans, have been eating meat, dairy products, and white bread for many years. Thus their biological constitution and their physiological functions are adapted to such foods. When they completely change to an Oriental diet - namely Macrobiotics - their digestive system may not function well. Many Orientals lived solely on rice and a few vegetables for many years. Rice is a highly nutritious food. It has proven to be so in the Orient. However, the number 7 diet (defined as grain and a little liquid) is perhaps fasting for many modern people, especially Americans, because in the beginning, they cannot assimilate its food value completely. (Fasting is a good remedy for many sicknesses, as stated in *Fasting Cure* by Upton Sinclair. However, fasting can sometimes cause very strong and drastic changes for modern Americans, especially those who have damaged their nervous system by long usage of drugs.)

Contrary to popular belief, the cause of Beth Ann Simon's death (see *The Macrobiotic*, Vol. II, #1 and #2) was that she and her husband were dabbling with not only Macrobiotics but also several other systems. They improved with Diet #7 but whenever leaving #7 they did so to an extreme. Diet #7 causes big changes in our body - namely Yangization (contraction, activation of the parasympathetic nerves, activation of the stomach, small intestines, large intestines, bladder, etc.). People are therefore attracted to strong yin (expansive) foods or liquid which stimulate the sympathetic nervous system, and in turn activate and yang organs such as heart, liver, kidney, and pancreas, and lead to exhaustion of these organs. This is the danger involved.

Most Americans today are too weak or sensitive in their nerve center - interbrain - which receives stimulation and sends out controlling messages to all organs, and any small change of the body's homeostasis can produce a big effect, and a swinging in between two extremes. For example, a small decrease of glucose in the blood (this is a yang condition) will cause a strong stimulation of the adrenalin gland which will produce much cortical hormone (this is a yin hormone) and change glycogen to glucose, causing the glucose level of the blood to become very high (this is a yin condition - the heart beat becomes faster, blood pressure rises). Then this high glucose level in turn stimulates the pancreas to produce insulin from the Islands of Langerhans. Insulin is a yang hormone which changes glucose to glycogen and stores it in the liver. As a result, the glucose level again goes down (a yang condition). Consequently, one swings from Yin to Yang, and Yang to Yin incessantly. One becomes more nervous. When he has a lower glucose level, he is attracted to sugar or fruit. Then he becomes more nervous and weak, and as a result, he is attracted to more yang foods - meat or salt. And after that he is attracted to more sweets. Such a vicious cycle is the danger involved.

We advise against a strict #7 diet for beginners for another reason also; the rigidity and fanaticism caused by fear. Most Americans have much fear, especially the sick. They read Ohsawa's books with fear of sickness. This word, #7 diet, can cause then to freeze - become rigid or fanatical. They lose their objectivity. They don't listen to other's warning or advice even when their sicknesses worsen. Mr. Ohsawa, therefore, warned them not to observe #7 blindly or without consulting him for a long period of time. But they will not see it. When they realize it, it may be too late.

Most Americans today, especially those who have been taking drugs have weak stomachs and intestines. Therefore, they cannot digest and assimilate their foods enough, especially brown rice which is quite strange to them. Since most of them have had meat-eating diets in the past, their system is adjusted to meat and not grains.

For the reasons mentioned, Americans should not start the Macrobiotic diet with a strict Regimen #7."

C. How to Start the Macrobiotic Diet

Read part "G" of the Appendix, "8 Principles of Macrobiotics" several times. It is not difficult to understand these principles conceptually, even though real understanding of them can take a lifetime. If you understand these principles, you will come to the idea that Macrobiotics is neither an exotic cuisine nor a restriction of what to eat. You must understand first that Macrobiotics is making order in eating. Man must have a man's order if he wants to establish a healthy condition and sane mentality. Sickness is nothing but a violation of man's order.

Macrobiotics teaches us how to establish and realize man's order in our daily life. The first step is to observe the first principle. Eat locally grown and seasonal grains and vegetables. This will eliminate all commercialized foods such as canned food, frozen food, tropical fruits, etc. Grains and seaweeds, however, can be eaten even though they come from foreign countries if they are not chemically treated (please see page 16 concerning seaweeds). The reason for this is that grains can be grown in most of the temperate zones. They have a very strong adaptability to the soil and climate changes.

The second step is to realize that whole foods are economical. Look for whole food in your neighborhood markets or health food stores. What are whole foods? That which are not refined, extracted, or made by synthetic chemicals. Therefore, refined flour, white bread, sugar, meat (this is only part of a cow), milk products (cream, cheese, etc. are part of milk), sugar products, etc. are not whole foods. All whole grains are whole foods. Small fish can be whole if you eat the head and tail. Eat vegetables, leaves, and roots. Whole foods contain all the nutrition and minerals needed. (Of course, some elements are contained in less quantity in certain foods than in others.) By eating whole foods, we will be able to maintain homeostasis and a good balance of nutrition in our blood, body fluid, and cells. By eating whole foods, we will be able to manufacture our own vitamins and enzymes. Therefore, by eating whole foods, we will be able to develop the ability of transmutation. When we acquire this, ability, we will be able to live on grains and vegetables, transmuting these to animal protein and body cells.

The third step is to apply the Yin-Yang principle in your selection of foods and cooking. However, don't be too nervous about the Yin and Yang of foods. If you follow the first step well, you are very well able to select foods from a Yin and Yang point of view. However, within the same shelf, you may be able to pick up a more yin or yang carrot, onion, or cabbage which suits your wishes. It is advisable to avoid tomato, egg plant, and potato, as they are extremely yin; due to longtime eating habits, however, those who crave these foods may eat them on occasion in small quantities. If you eat a small quantity, you can eat anything without any harm. Don't restrict yourself because this creates a reaction of extreme bingeing.

The fourth step is to learn cooking techniques that change yin foods to yang ones, and make foods more delicious. Heat, pressure, salt and time (ageing) are the magicians for the yangization of foods. For yang foods, one of these techniques may be enough. However, yin foods may require three or more of these processes of yangization. For example, yang burdock requires heat and salt in cooking, whereas yin soybeans require heat, pressure, salt, and time. Traditional Japanese foods and condiments, which are artistic and nutritious products, apply these techniques to yin foods.

Applying the Yin-Yang principle; your cooking attitude, selection of foods, and delicacy of taste will improve tremendously. You will no longer be a mere cook, but an artist or creator of life. When you can bring more joy and happiness to your dinner table, your Macrobiotic diet is on the way.

26

In hot weather, climates or location, or with very yang foods, we use the opposite technique - yinization; that is to say, use of vinegar, wine, ginger, spices, raw vegetables and fermentation. For example, we add grated radish to fish, or fried vegetables (tempura). Green leaves are added to raw fish (Sashimi). Yinization is also the technique applied to food that is to be eaten by a very yang person.

This principle leads us to a higher technique of cooking - the combination of foods. When you master this you are the master of cooking. You can originate your own delicious recipes which will surprise your guest whenever he visits you.

The fifth step is learning the application of the principle of transmutation. In other words, avoid foods which will not require thorough use of our digestion or transmutation function.

Milk and milk products are such a food. No animal gives milk after their baby is grown except man. Milk is the proper food for a baby who is not able to digest and transmute grains and vegetables for their own nutrition, because milk is very easy to change into blood, body energy and cells. Therefore, one raised on milk will not develop much ability to transmute and will be upset easily when brought into contact with a foreign food or matter. An allergic constitution is the result. Such a person cannot transmute foreign food, or foreign ideas to his own. He must live in a small world exclusively. It is a pity that he cannot embrace everything. Even though he may build a cow's body, he cannot create a thousand friends all over the world.

The sixth step is learning to plan the menu wisely. The following percentages are approximations. Each individual must carefully consider his previous eating habits, amount and type of activity, age, climatic conditions, season of the year, etc. In order to determine his needs at any particular time, keeping in mind that his needs will change as his condition changes:

	Winter cold climate	Fall/Spring temperate climate	Summer hot climate
Grains	70-90	50-70	30-50
Vegetables	10-30	30-50	50-70
Beans	5-10	7-12	10-15
Seaweeds	5-10	7-12	10-15
Pressed salad	5-10	7-12	10-15
Fish	10	5	2

Raw vegetables, cooked fruit, nuts, and dairy products are eaten on occasion and sometimes are even recommended. All foods used should be in season (fresh), locally grown, and free of all synthetic chemicals (preservatives, sprays, dyes, etc) Vitamin pills (whether natural or synthetic) and 'enriched' foods should also be completely avoided.

The following is a possible basic menu, chosen for its simplicity, which is ideal for a single person or family, new to Macrobiotics where cooking skills are limited. Vary the meals to suit yourself. Recipes can be found on the following pages, or in *Cooking Good Foods, Cooking With Grains*, etc. For more diversified recipes, see *Zen Macrobiotic Cooking* and *Cooking for Life* by Michel Abehsera.

Breakfast: Rice cream, Wheat cream or Rolled oats

Whole grain bread (optional)

Cup of Miso/Wakame soup (optional) with or without fish (small dried fish)

(Miso soup is listed here with every meal as optional, however it is suggested that it be served only once a day, at whichever meal is preferred.)

Pressed salad

Tea (not dyed)

Lunch:
Rice or another grain (barley is good in the summer, wheat, buckwheat - winter only because it is very yang), etc. or a combination such as rice and wheat, rice and barley, aduki/rice, etc. Try them all.

Vegetables (any except tomatoes, potatoes, and eggplant), sauteed, pressure-cooked, baked, tempura, etc. They can be prepared in large quantities and used for two or three days.

Beans (aduki, chickpeas, lentils, black beans, etc.) You can prepare enough for a few days at a time. (Good with sauteed onions.)

Whole grain bread (optional)

Miso soup (optional)

Pressed salad

Tea

Supper:
Rice (or another grain) and/or noodles (whole-wheat, buckwheat, Udon, etc.)

Vegetables

Hiziki (a kind of seaweed; it can be prepared for a few days at a time.) As cooking skill improves, try others; nori, kombu, wakame, dulse, etc. In winter, Hiziki is very good with lotus root or burdock.

Beans

Whole grain bread (optional)

Miso soup (optional)

Pressed salad

Fish (optional)

29

Tea (one who doesn't want tea or water after every meal is too yin. Either he is not getting enough exercise or his food is too yin.)

Some people may want to skip breakfast or substitute lunch for breakfast and skip lunch. This is recommended for people having trouble with over-eating. If you eat only twice a day you can eat a larger amount each time. This often helps to keep the total daily intake lower.

Fish flakes and/or Chuba Iriko (small whole fishes) can be used in soup or other cooking on a daily basis, if desired. When using them you will need considerably less or no salt. In hot weather you can completely eliminate all fish in most cases

Until very recently, Japanese people very rarely ate desserts as we know them (including cooked fruit). Instead, they considered mochi (paddled rice cakes, plain, with aduki beans or other fillings) and/or pressed salad to be dessert. You are urged to do likewise.

For the first few days or weeks of observing the Macrobiotic diet it may be difficult to eliminate sweets. For this reason, small amounts of raw fruit or even honey can be used, especially when eating fish at the same meal. Sugar should be eliminated, however, in the beginning; honey should be eliminated as soon as possible, and raw fruits should generally be taken only in hot weather or by those who have much stored-up animal protein. Desserts made with cooked nuts, raisins, or chestnuts (cookies, pies, etc.) baked apples, etc. can be eaten often, depending on climate, season, constitutional condition and age. They should be given more often to children than to adults.

Some people have a lot of difficulty avoiding taking sugar even after several years. If this is true in your case, eat more pumpkin, squash (especially brown varieties such as acorn or butternut) and aduki beans. Pumpkin and squash are very sweet, especially when baked. If you are still having difficulty, try some cooked or raw fruit in small amounts. In any case, it is better to avoid tropical fruit in this climatic zone.

Pressed salad and/or pickles can be served at every meal. We have found them to be very helpful in maintaining a consistent diet. Also, if you suddenly find yourself becoming too yang, rather than drinking a pot of tea, greedily devouring one or two raw apples, or frantically gulping tap water, take some pressed salad instead. Or, if there is none available, try some raw carrot, lettuce, white radish, cabbage, red radish, or cucumber.

Pickles and Pressed Salad:

1. Place in a keg - most yang method: (a) Dried fresh daikon (white radish): place alternative layers of (1) a mixture of 15-20 cups of rice bran and 2-3 cups of sea salt, and (2) about 50 large whole daikon (about the size of carrots - these are the daikon which are harvested in late fall and winter, as opposed to the smaller variety, which are harvested all year around and are not suitable for this recipe) which have been kept from rain and hung outside to dry for about two weeks in a clean, dry keg with a wooden cover directly on top of the last layer of daikon. The cover must be small enough so that it will sink as the water rises and excess is removed from the keg (to be used in soups or other cooking). On top of the cover, place a heavy rock. After about 10 days, put in a cool place and remove excess liquid. These will be ready in one or two months, and will last about 4 months. (The longer you want the pickles to last, the more salt you will need.)
(b) Un-dried daikon pickles: same procedure, but use less salt. Ready in about 2-3 weeks, and will last about three months. (Less salt is needed with undried daikon because the salt will react more quickly when the daikon are not dried.)
(c) Pickles made from other vegetables: (chopped or separated cabbage, Chinese cabbage, celery, lettuce, cucumbers, etc.); these are not dried first. Instead of the rice-bran and salt mixture, use plain salt - about 15 lbs. of vegetables to 1 cup sea salt. These are ready in about

31

3 days, and will last about 2-3 months if kept in a cool place.

2. In a salad press - more yin: Chop vegetables. Use about ½ Tbls. salt to ½ cabbage or an equivalent amount of other vegetables. Mix together and put in the press. Tighten. When liquid is expelled, tighten press, but leave liquid (to allow salt, which will be absorbed in liquid, to yangize the vegetables. Tighten from time to time. These can be eaten after a few hours, but they taste better after one or two days.

3. In a hurry: Chop vegetables. Add a little salt. Squeeze in hands. (This is the most yin of the three methods; pressure, time, and salt are yang.)

There are several reasons why most Americans starting the Macrobiotic diet should take only small amounts of salt. First, since salt is very yang, it holds Yin in the body, restraining its expulsion. Second, excess salt leads to over-eating or bingeing. Third, it is impossible to yangize quickly without later going in the opposite direction at a similar speed. Fourth, most of us have a long history of meat-eating and are thus able to take much less salt than Orientals. (In fact, because of the meat, Westerners have much more salt stock than Orientals.) Fifth, most youth of America today are lazy and don't work. Therefore, they can't take salt (and therefore can't work).

To avoid eating sugar and bingeing, one should eat less extreme yang foods, such as burdock, Kuzu, buckwheat, millet, fish, fowl, salt, or mu tea. Another way is by taking slightly more yin foods, such as vegetables, yin grains, raw vegetables, cooked beans, or seaweeds (kombu and wakame can be eaten raw). A third way to avoid extremes is by activity. When one has a weak inter-brain, his nervous system is too sensitive to stimulation. As a result, the nervous system over-acts and creates the attraction of extremes. To strengthen the inter-brain, one should keep a little hungry all the time, be active at anything or do hard physical work. Give constantly your service and smile to others; hard work is good medicine, even when one is weak.

A Simple Meal:
Rice
Vegetable
Miso Soup

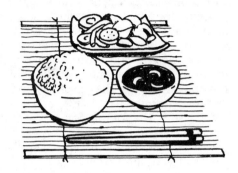

D. Macrobiotic Cooking

1. What is Macrobiotic cooking?

Nature gives man everything - Yin and Yang - sunshine and water, rain, breeze and storm, ocean and mountain, ice, clouds, hot and cold, desert and flood, disease and health, war and peace, bitter and sour, hot and cool, salty and sweet. Man is born in this world naked and unfree. He would die immediately not having protection of shelter, care of mother, milk for food. However, he is destined to become the freest creature on the earth, receiving all kinds of natural trials and human education. In order to reach human faculties, he must develop his most precise machine - the human body - up to the point that he can maintain homeostatic internal conditions which are constant under any outside changes. He must develop his amazing nervous and hormonal system so that he can maintain orderly activities of various organs. He must develop his inter-brain so that he can maintain his calmness and elegance in a storm, lightning, flood, war, desperation, hostility and all trials. He must develop his brain so that he can enjoy the humor of Mark Twain, simplicity of Haiku, greatness in a small flower, and usefulness in no use.

Furthermore, he must transmute everything as he wishes. Vegetables to animals, carbohydrates to sugar, sugar to protein, sodium to potassium, magnesium to iron, foods to blood, bitterness to sweet, anger to joy, anxiety to peace, jealousy to generosity, exclusivity to all-embracement, and arrogance to humility. The ability of this transmutation is the freedom which all men wish to acquire. Such freedom is possible when one has healthy body fluids, organs, nervous systems, hormonal systems, and brains. Man's physiological condition is the foundation of the freedom of transmutation.

Such freedom of transmutation will be developed by daily practice - especially in eating and drinking. The discipline toward freedom of transmutation is the Macrobiotic diet, and the preparation of the diet is Macrobiotic cooking.

Cooking makes our transmutation easier, faster and smoother. Without proper cooking man will have many difficulties in assimilating and digesting some of the foods he eats, in maintaining his homeostatic internal conditions, and in maintaining a healthy and happy mentality among ever challenging stress and strain. In other words, cooking is not merely the technique to make delicious cuisines but it is also a sacred ceremony where nature and human action meet. Foods are the principal elements of life. The kitchen is the studio where life is created. Cooking must be performed by an artist's sense, a scientist's precision and a philosopher's deep understanding.

Macrobiotic cooking is a life long study and discipline which man cannot forget even for a day. Macrobiotic cooking is the source of a strong body and high judgment, without which man can never be happy and free.

2. The way of Macrobiotic cooking.

Macrobiotic cooking is nothing but the application of the Order of Nature which is that everything changes - Yin to Yang, Yang to Yin. Cooking is a technique that promotes this change so that man can establish the order of Man within himself. In other words, cooking brings him order of body fluids, organs, the nervous system and brain. Some foods, however, are too far away from this order. Some foods are not suited to man. Therefore, the first step of cooking is the selection of foods.

3. The selection of foods.

There are thousands of kinds of foods on the earth. We can divide them into two - one is animal foods and the other is vegetal foods. We use mostly vegetal foods because animals are the terminus of evolution of life. (Life is a spiralic transmutation starting from Oneness to the animal world.) Animal is the end stage of this evolution of life. Its next step is decomposition. Therefore, if our diet consists chiefly of animal foods, our body decomposes - a cancerous condition.

Vegetal foods, contrary to animal foods, are an immature stage of life. They are virgin life. Therefore, vegetal foods create our body, rejuvenate us and make us healthy.

There is an order in the selection of vegetal foods. The first choice is grains because grains are the most abundant vegetables and our tooth structure tells us that we are grain eaters. Next to grain is vegetables - mountain, field and ocean vegetables. The rough food order for man should be as follows: grains, vegetables, salt, oil, fish, nuts, fruits, milk, meat, eggs, spices (see *The Macrobiotic*, Vol. 10, #4).

In order to select our foods further, we use three principles: ecology of life, economy of life, and the Yin-Yang principle. In short, follow the order of space and time. Select the foods which grow nearest your environment. Cook the foods as whole as possible, so that you will get whole nutrition. Whole foods have life; partial food does not. Life contains whole nutrition because it is living. However, the part of a food is not living and therefore it is not complete nutrition. For example, we use carrot leaves for tempura instead of throwing them away. This is the same as for scallion roots, and others. Don't skin off lotus root or burdock root. We use fish head for soup stock. He who makes much waste is not a good cook.

Balancing is important in selection of foods. Use land vegetables with ocean vegetables. Add vegetables to animal foods. Potassium rich foods must be balanced by heat, pressure and salt, because the first is yin and the latter is yang.

4. Cutting.
Vegetables must be washed gently, eliminating dirt and spoiled parts. Don't crush the leaves when you wash them. Cutting is determined by the type of cuisine. If you cook stew or nitsuke which require longer cooking, cut them in larger sizes. However, when cooking in a hurry, cut them thin so that they can cook in a short time. It is better to cut small and thin pieces for miso soup. Cut in large pieces for Russian soup, stew and oden (Japanese vegetable stew with authentic soy sauce).

Thought must be given to the Yin-Yang balance of vegetables when cutting them. For example, cutting an onion horizontally makes yang onion and yin onion, meaning that some will get only yin parts and some will get only yang parts. You must, therefore, cut an onion vertically, turning it at its axis, so that every piece will contain Yin and Yang. The top part of the root is more yin than the bottom. Cutting diagonally to include the ends will create a good balance of Yin and Yang. The shape of vegetables make a cuisine beautiful and attractive. Insensitive cutting spoils the delicacy and taste of the cuisine. Also, the cutting board and knife must be cleaned whenever different vegetables are cut because it keeps Yin and Yang in the right order.

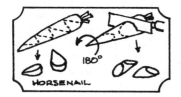

HORSENAIL

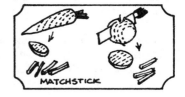

MATCHSTICK

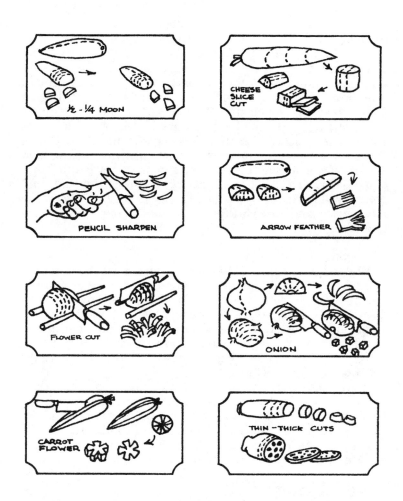

5. Cooking.

Do not use sugar or mono-sodium-glutamate. This is the first rule of cooking. The distinctive taste of each food must be fully introduced in the cuisine and yet when finished they are well blended as a whole. There are seven ways of cooking: boiling, baking, broiling, pressure-cooking, sauteeing, frying, steaming. Begin foods first that require longer cooking time.

In cooking, orderliness must be observed. Clothes and appearance must be neat and orderly and all finished pans must be cleaned right away and made ready for the next use. The order of cooking must be figured out before starting to cook; otherwise, much time will be wasted. Such orderliness is important in cooking because it makes less waste, mistakes and at the end, a better taste and greater nutritional value will result. One's character is reflected in his cooking and cuisine. For example, a careless person produces cooking that is very disorderly. On the contrary, a thoughtful and kind person will make satisfying and wholesome dishes. Therefore, love, giving and thoughtfulness are the fundamental principles of cooking.

6. Serving.

Moderation, neatness and balance concerning the foods are important. Normally, grains should represent 50% or more of the diet. On some occasions or for beginners, however, side dishes can be increased. The combination of foods, shapes, colors and tastes must be well arranged. For example, grated radish with mochi, grated radish and parsley, or sliced radish for tempura or sashimi are good combinations. Ginger always enhances the taste of fish.

Yang foods must be combined with yin foods. Yin foods must be combined with yang foods. For example, salmon head is good cooked with soybeans. Lotus root and hijiki, azuki and kombu, radish and fish are good combinations.

Do not mix hot and cold foods in a lunch box because such mixing will cause fermentation.

7. General suggestions.

Prepare, cook and serve with care and love. Love and care make the difference in taste and appearance and is the key to success in cooking. Only with love and care is your cooking creative, unique and wholesome.

Setting the dinner table is the joyful ritual of the family and a place to show gratitude. In such a family, there will be no room for sickness and agony.

As a last suggestion, hunger is the best seasoning of any dishes. One day, the Zen monk Takuan invited a lord to his temple for dinner. The lord waited and waited many hours expecting Takuan to serve him a delicious meal. Hours later, however, Takuan served him brown rice and radish pickles. It was the most delicious meal the lord had ever had, because he was so hungry after waiting for such a long time.

Chew well and eat moderately. These are the best manners at the dinner table.

8. Cooking summary.

    a. Main foods: Grains - brown rice, buckwheat, wheat, millet and barley, rye, oats, and corn.

    b. Secondary foods: Vegetables in season - 1/3 of food intake. Seaweeds, beans - 1/3 of vegetables. The rest will be fish, eggs, milk, nuts, fruits, seeds, milk products, fowl.

    c. Seasoning: salt, oil, authentic soy sauce, miso.

    d. Use whole foods. Waste nothing.

    e. Products from far away places and different seasons should be avoided. White rice, white bread, meat, sugar, candy, foreign fruits, chemical additives, chemical products, chemical seasonings are not conducive to good health. They should generally be avoided.

    f. Chew well.

    g. Eat radish pickles or miso pickles after cleaning the bowl with them. In this way, Zen monks saved cleaning time of dishes.

    h. A little sesame salt, shio-kombu, kimpira, or tekka can be served at every meal.

i. Make your own pickles all the time so that you can make varieties in dishes and can do a good service to your unexpected friends.

j. For busy people, cook for a week and store food in the refrigerator. Miso soup cannot be kept more than a few days because the taste deteriorates, so store the soup stock and add miso fresh at each heating.

E. Recipes.

1. Cooked Brown Rice:

   a. Pressure cooked
      1 cup brown rice (serves 2)
      1¼ cup water
      ¼ tsp. salt
      Wash rice gently until water is clear. Put measured water and rice into a pressure cooker. If your pressure cooker is old and steam escapes out the sides and strong pressure is not created when food is cooked in it, soak the rice overnight. Add salt just before cooking, cover and cook on low heat for 30 minutes, then turn to "high" until pressure comes up full. Lower heat and cook 45-60 minutes. Turn off heat and allow pressure to return to normal. Let stand for 20-30 minutes. Remove cover and mix rice thoroughly before serving.

   b. Boiled rice
      4 cups rice (serves 7)
      6-7 cups water
      1 tsp. salt
      Wash rice as in (a). Add salt just before cooking. Cook on low heat for 30 minutes, then turn heat to "high" until boiling. After this, cook rice on medium heat for 20 minutes and then 40 minutes on low heat. Turn heat off and allow cooked rice to sit for 40 minutes. Remove cover and mix thoroughly before serving.

2. Creamed Onion-Miso Soup:
   6 small whole onions
   2 carrots cut on the diagonal in ¼" thick slices
   ½ tsp. salt
   ½ cup wholewheat pastry flour
   2 tsp. oil
   6 cups water
   3 Tbsp. Miso (soybean paste)

   Heat oil, add whole onions and saute a few minutes.
   Then add carrots and saute also for a few minutes. Add
   2 cups water and salt and pressure cook vegetables for 5
   to 7 minutes. Saute flour in 2 tsp. oil until it is slightly
   darkened in color and has a nut-like fragrance. Stir
   constantly while roasting. Cool, then make a paste of
   the roasted flour by adding cold water. After pressure
   has gone down, add 4 cups water to the cooked onion
   and carrots and bring to a boil. Add the above flour
   paste mixture to the soup to thicken it. Add the Miso
   soybean paste and cook for a few minutes. Serve with
   minced parsley on top.

3. Tempura:

   Vegetables are dipped or mixed with batter and deep
   fried in corn oil or a mixture of corn and sesame oil.
   The vegetables and the batter should be chilled. For best
   results mix batter just prior to use. The oil should be 3"
   deep and heated to approximately 350 degrees. When
   the batter-dipped vegetables are added to the oil they
   should fall to the bottom of the pan and almost
   immediately pop to the surface. When the top side of
   each piece turns yellow, turn over and cook until each
   piece is tan colored. In deep frying, one heaping
   teaspoon of the vegetable mixture should be put in at a
   time. There should be no more than one line of tempura
   pieces covering the oil in the pan at one time. If the
   batter disperses a little bit in the oil, usually this makes
   good tempura. However, if the batter does not disperse
   when placed in the oil, then it is too heavy so add a

little bit of water. Drain each tempura piece well by placing in a strainer which has been set on a bowl to catch the excess oil. Then after draining, set the pieces on paper toweling and serve hot.

Batter for Tempura

1 cup wholewheat pastry flour
1¼ cup water
½ tsp. salt
1 heaping tsp. corn starch

Add ½ of the water to dry ingredients, mix; then add rest of water, mixing lightly. It doesn't matter if the batter is lumpy.

Variations of Tempura

Carrot:
Cut carrots on the diagonal in ¼" thick slices. Mix with sufficient amount of batter and deep fry in oil.

Onion:
Cut onions in half lengthwise and slice thinly, leaving a piece of hard core at the bottom to hold the slivers together. Each piece should look like a fan. Dip into batter and deep fry.

Watercress:
Leave whole, dip in batter and deep fry.

Cauliflower:
Break into flowerettes, dip in batter and deep fry.

Squash or pumpkin:
Cut in 1" wide x 3" long and ¼" thick pieces. Dip in batter and deep fry.

Sweet potato:
Cut on the diagonal in ½" thick pieces. Dip in batter and deep fry.

Corn (fresh):
Scrape kernels off cob. Add chopped onions and mix with batter. Drop by spoonfuls into deep oil.

Any of these vegetables can be used in combinations with one another. Serve with grated daikon radish mixed with authentic soy sauce for easy digestion or with tempura sauce with grated radish.

Tempura Sauce

>1 cup kombu soup stock
>2 Tbsp. authentic soy sauce

>Bring the above mixture to a boil.

Kombu soup stock

>16 cups water
>3" x 12" kombu (dashi kombu seaweed found in
>   Japanese food stores)
>¾ cup chuba iriko (dried Japanese fish)

>Cut 12" long piece of kombu using a scissor into 1" thick slices leaving ½" attached to one side. Do not cut all the way through. See diagram:

>Place kombu (may be cut in half into 6" long pieces) in 8 cups of water. Bring to boil with cover. Add fish and boil again without cover. Drain off liquid into a bowl. Reserve kombu and fish. Add 8 more cups of water, bring to boil and cook 30 minutes with cover on. Drain and mix with first stock or use separately, since they have a slightly different taste.

4. Stuffed Cabbage with Carrot Roll:

>Carrot Rolls (makes 40 rectangular rolls)
>2 cups finely grated carrots
>1 cup minced onion
>2 cups wholewheat flour
>½ cup buckwheat flour
>2 tsp. salt

>Mix all ingredients together. Form into ½" x 2"

rectangular shapes and deep fry until brown and crispy in 350 degrees oil. These rolls can be used in other dishes - shaped in ball form - such as in chop suey, cauliflower gratin, or with vegetables and kuzu arrowroot sauce.

Take cabbage out of refrigerator and allow to sit at room temperature for half a day. Take all leaves off gently and wash. In salted water boil leaves a few minutes until they change to a greener color. Take out of water and put in a strainer. Cut off a 1" triangle from the hard white part of each leaf. Place one carrot roll on each cabbage leaf and wrap inside like a package. First fold over the hard white part of the leaf to cover the carrot roll, then fold over the two sides of the leaf and roll. Insert a toothpick to hold the leaf together. Follow the same procedure for the rest of the cabbage leaves and carrot rolls. Set all stuffed cabbage rolls in pan covered with water and bring to a boil. Cook 20 minutes. Add 1 tsp. salt and 2 tsp. authentic soy sauce and cook 10 more minutes.

White Sauce

Heat fry pan, then add 1 tbsp. oil and heat to boiling. Add 1 cup unbleached white flour. Roast on a medium flame and keep stirring for 5 minutes. When color is slightly changed (not brown) turn off heat and allow flour to cool. Then add 3-4 cups water, mix together and bring to a boil. Add ½ tsp. salt and cook at boiling point for 5 minutes. Cover cabbage rolls with this sauce. Boil a few minutes and serve. (This sauce can be served over deep-fried carrot balls as a dish also.)

5. Wholewheat Spaghetti Gratin with Salmon:

> 1½ packages wholewheat spaghetti
> 2 small onions sliced thinly
> 3 cabbage leaves - cut thinly in 1½" lengths
> 2 celery stalks (cut thinly on the diagonal)
> 1 piece baked and chopped salmon
> 1 tsp. oil
> 2 tsp. salt

After water comes to a boil add salt and spaghetti, cover and bring to a boil again. After boiling add 2 cups cold water, mixing in from top to bottom. Cover and bring again to a boil. Then shut off heat and let stand with cover on for a few minutes. Test spaghetti by placing one strand in a bowl of cold water. Cut and if color is the same inside and outside, the spaghetti is done. Wholewheat spaghetti takes longer to cook than regular white spaghetti, so allow for this. Drain and rinse noodles with cold water a couple of times until they become cool. If noodles are not rinsed they later become very soft. (The salted water used in cooking the spaghetti can be reserved and used in soup or for the liquid in bread-making.)

Bechamel Sauce

> ½ cup wholewheat pastry flour
> 1 tsp. salt
> 1 Tbsp. oil
> 2½ cups water

Heat the oil slightly, add the flour gently and roast, stirring constantly. Do not roast too long - only until the lumps disappear. Allow the flour to turn color slightly. For the best results cool. Add water and boil for 5 minutes, stirring occasionally. Add salt and simmer for 15 minutes longer. Set aside.

In another pan heat oil, saute onions until they are transparent, add cabbage and saute until their color is changed. Add celery and saute a few minutes longer.

Then add salt and cook until partly tender. Put cooked spaghetti in a covered casserole with vegetables on top. Crumble the salmon over this and cover with the bechamel sauce. Bake 20-30 minutes in a 350 degree oven.

6. Chickpeas with Sauce:

1 cup chickpeas
1 medium onion
1 tsp. oil
2 cups water

Soak chickpeas overnight in 2 cups of water. Mince onion, saute in oil until light brown in color. (Saute the onion in a pressure cooker pan.) Add chickpeas and soaking water and cover. Bring pressure up by turning heat on "high" and after the pressure cooker top is jiggling, turn heat to "low" and cook 45 minutes. Turn off heat and allow pressure to come down.

Sauce

1 cup sliced onion - cut in 8 pieces
3 cups cauliflower - cut in flowerettes
½ cup carrot slices - cut carrots in half lengthwise and then on the diagonal in ¼" thick slices
2 tsp. oil
2 tsp. salt
2 tsp. tahini (sesame butter found in health food stores or Greek food stores.)

Heat pan, add oil and heat to boiling. Add onions and saute until transparent. Add cauliflower and saute 5 minutes then add carrot and saute a few minutes. Add water and cover vegetables. Bring to a boil and then simmer 20 minutes. Add chickpeas (and the water they have been cooked in) to the vegetables and cook 20 minutes. To this add salt and cook 15 minutes more. Add tahini and cook 5 minutes. Gently mix the vegetables and tahini. Serve hot over rice or on bread.

7. Romaine Lettuce Pressed Salad:

>2 heads Romaine lettuce
>1 carrot cut very thinly like matchsticks
>½ bunch red radishes cut in thin rounds
>2 tsp. salt
>3 bunches scallions cut very thinly

Cut lettuce in quarters, open and cut in 1" pieces. Mix all ingredients thoroughly with the salt. Place in a Japanese vegetable press or in a bowl with a plate pressing the salad and a heavy object such as a rock on top of the plate. When the water comes out and to the top, pour it off, leaving at least ½" so that the salad will not spoil. The salad can then be eaten, but it is more delicious if kept 2-3 days before eating. In the winter it is best this way.

8. Apple Crisp:

>4 cups sliced apples or peaches in season
>1/3 cup wholewheat flour
>1 cup uncooked rolled oats
>½ tsp. salt
>1 tsp. cinnamon
>1 tsp. grated lemon rind
>1/8 cup water and 1/8 cup oil mixed together

Place apples in an oiled shallow baking dish, sprinkle with lemon rind. Combine dry ingredients. Add oil mixing until crumbly. Sprinkle crumb mixture over apples. Bake in a 350 degree oven for 30 minutes or until apples are tender.

F. Does the Macrobiotic Diet Supply Enough Protein?

In the latter half of the 19th century, Voit suggested that the protein requirement for the average person is 118 g. and 145 g. for the heavy laborer. An American nutritionist, Atwater, recommended 125 g. which was the standard requirement of protein for several decades. McCay in 1912 concluded in his study that the amount of protein contained in the food contributes to a higher grade of muscle strength, durability, resistance to diseases, courage and fighting spirit. In other words, a race that consumes more animal protein is stronger and more manly.

However, in 1901, Russell Chittenden of Yale University claimed that the protein requirement should be reduced to 2/3. Horace Fletcher - of "Fletcherism" - observed a diet under the supervision of Dr. Chittenden consisting of 43 g. of protein for several months and maintained 75 kg. of weight. He could even do heavy activity.

Chittenden did further experiments with 5 teachers, 13 soldiers and 8 athletes and analyzed their intake and excretions for 225 days. Chittenden concluded that one is able to maintain good health by consuming 36 g. of protein and 2000 calories of food energy daily. He maintained his weight at 125 lbs. Dr. Mendel maintained good health at 154 lbs. with a daily consumption of 40 g. of protein. All the others also maintained good health on the low protein diet.

Chittenden concluded that:

1. Protein cannot be stored in our body tissue.
2. Our body will waste energy with excess protein.
3. Excess protein will create toxins by fermentation in the large intestine.
4. Protein is not necessary as an energy source because carbohydrates and fats can do the job efficiently.
5. It is necessary to take animal and vegetable protein in good proportion.

Today the scientists differ in their opinions on the amount of protein required for good health. According to the report of the World Health Organization, the requirements of protein for the average adult is 0.59 grams per kilogram of body weight per day. If one person weighs about 130 lbs. he must take 36 g. of protein per day.

According to "Composition of Foods" by the U.S. Department of Agriculture, 1 lb. of each of these foods contains the following amount of protein:

Abalone	35 g	Almond	43 g	Apple	.8 g
Bacon	38	Barley	37	Black sea bass	34
Striped bass	37	Lima beans	38	Beef	53
T-bone steak	59.1	Bread	40	Buttermilk	16
Cheese	80-100	Cottage cheese	60	Chicken	40
Corn meal	40	Sweet corn	8	Corn flour	35
Clam meat	60	Crab meat	75	Chicken egg	58
Egg yolk	49	Egg white	72	Halibut	56
Macaroni	56	Milk	16	Oatmeal	64
Oyster meat	38	Pork	32.6	Rice	34
Rye	55	Salmon	66	Sesame seed	84.4
Soybeans - mature/dry	154	Natto	76.7	Miso	47.6
Soy sauce	25	Spaghetti	57	Trout	97
Tuna meat	114	Turkey	50	Veal	66
Wheat - whole grain	64	Flour	60		

1 lb. of rice will supply enough protein for the average adult per day; 10 oz. of Miso will be enough. Therefore, 8 oz. of rice, 1 oz. of Miso, soy sauce, 2 oz. of beans, seaweed and some pieces of bread will supply enough protein for average Americans.

Soybeans and sesame seeds have almost all the amino acids. Therefore, Miso, authentic soy sauce, and sesame salt are some of the best condiments. If these are used daily with grains and vegetables, the supply of essential amino acids will be enough, provided that one is able to assimilate those nutrients.

According to modern nutrition theories, there are 8-10 essential amino acids which must be supplied by the foods we eat. They are:

	Cow	Pig	Soybean	Sesame Seeds
Tryptophan	.073	.081	.086	.091
Threonine	.276	.290	.246	.194
Isoleucine	.327	.321	.336	.261
Leucine	.572	.460	.482	.461
Lysine	.546	.460	.395	.160
Methionine	.155	.156	.084	.175
Thistine	.079	.073	.111	.136
Phenylanine	.257	.246	.309	.400
Tyrosine	.212	.223	.199	.261
Valine	.347	.325	.328	.244

This table shows the amount of essential amino acids per gram in proportion to each 1 g. of nitrogen in the foods according to *Importance of Vegetarianism* by Dr. M. Ushio.

Underlined numbers show the highest amount of essential amino acids within these four foods. Animal foods contain the highest amount of 4 essential amino acids; threonine, leucine, lysine, and valine. Vegetable foods, however, contain the highest amount of 6 essential amino acids: tryptophan, isoleucine, thistine, phenylalanine, tyrosine, and methionine.

Lysine and leucine which have a high content in animal foods are related to growth. Therefore, adults who have stopped growing do not need much of these amino acids. Tryptophan and thistine are related to the maintenance and metabolism of the body. Therefore, these are preferable for grown-ups. This comparison, however, does not recommend a meat diet for the young, because children can transmute their own protein from carbohydrates. In contrast to the commonly accepted theory, we recommend less animal food for children after nursing. Many children are quite healthy without meat and fish, although they are not as husky as meat-fed children.

The food value of protein from different sources in terms of their essential amino acid composition (mg of amino acid/g of nitrogen - from *Man and Food* by Magnus Pyke) is shown in Table A, on the following page.

Dr. Bieler in his *Food is Your Best Medicine* warns that excess animal protein can be harmful to us. We agree with him on this point. Animal protein should be eaten moderately. At the beginning of Macrobiotics, fish or fowl can be eaten 3-4 times a week; 3 months later, 2-3 times a week; 1 year later, once a week; three years after starting the diet, fish or fowl can be eaten according to desire, weather, and activity. One who does much physical work may have more than one who does less physical work. At the beginning, if you crave meat, you may eat it instead of fish or fowl. However, go back to the other as soon as possible.

Table A

	Ideal Protein	Egg	Meat (Beef)	Milk (Cow's)	Fish	Oats	Rice	Flour (White)
Isoleucine	270	428	332	407	317	302	312	262
Leucine	306	565	575	630	474	436	535	442
Lysine	270	396	540	496	549	212	236	126
Phenylanine	180	368	256	311	231	309	307	322
Tyrosine	180	274	212	323	159	213	269	174
Methionine	144	196	154	154	178	84	142	78
Threonine	180	310	275	292	283	192	241	174
Tryptophan	90	106	75	90	62	74	65	69
Valine	270	460	345	440	327	348	415	262
Score	100	100	83	78	70	79	72	47

G. Vitamins

Next to wondering if one gets the necessary amount of protein in a Macrobiotic diet, the question most often asked is whether or not there is too much cooking involved. Does not the cooking destroy vitamins? I have written about the principle of cooking in the previous chapter. Here I will explain about vitamins.

History of Vitamins:

The cause of scurvy has been considered as a deficiency of nutrients for many years. The first race that discovered the cure for scurvy was the Canadian Indian as reported by Biggar in 1924. They had suffered from this disease every winter until they found the cure by eating pine leaves. By applying this finding, Jacques Cartier produced good results

51

when some of his expedition members suffered from scurvy at the bank of the St. Lawrence River. James Lind (1753) cured the sailors of scurvy by giving them oranges and lemons.

Around 1880, Japanese navy sailors suffered from beri-beri. Admiral K. Takagi changed their diet, adding more meat and vegetables. This lessened the occurrence of the disease.

Eijkman, in 1897, experimentally produced beri-beri, which was common in rice-eating people, in chickens by giving them white rice. He also found that it can be prevented by giving whole brown rice. However, he could not explain the reason for this.

In 1911, the Polish chemist Casimir Funk succeeded in extracting from rice polishings a crystaline substance which, in fact, cured beri-beri. This is now called Vitamin B_1 or Thiamine.

When analyzed, these crystals revealed the presence of nitrogen in basic combination; that is, the so-called "amine nitrogen". Therefore, Funk coined the word "vitamine" as the name of this life-giving substance from the prefix "vita", meaning "life", and the suffix "amine". Thus the word vitamine was born. The revised spelling "vitamin" was adopted to indicate that most of these compounds are not amines.

Kinds of Vitamins:

There are many vitamins. Each authority lists a different number. Professional nutrition books list large numbers of vitamins and some have more than one name. For example, the Vitamin B complex is made up of many vitamins. Niacin is also called nicotinic acid; B_1 is thiamine; B_2 is riboflavin or G; B_6 is pyridoxine; B_{12} is cobalancin. There are also B_3, B_{15}, and B_{17}. Parts of the B complex are biotin (called H), choline, inositol, folic or folinic acid, pantothenic acid, para-aminobenzoic acid and B-t (called carnitine). There is A, C, or ascorbic acid with the bioflavinoids formerly called P, D_1, D_2, D_3, E, F (the unsaturated fatty acids), G, or riboflavin, as was stated, H, or biotin as above, K_1, K_2, and many other chemical names for these same vitamins. Furthermore, it is probable that many more vitamins will be discovered in the years to come.

Characteristics of Vitamins:
1. Vitamin C - Please read *Vitamin C and Fruit* by Henaff and George Ohsawa - a GOMF publication.

The chief sources of Vitamin C are citrus fruits, tomatoes, and leafy vegetables, preferably raw. There are smaller amounts in all other fruits and vegetables. This indicates that Vitamin C is yin. Vitamin C is decomposed when heated - a Yin indication. When seeds, grains, and legumes are sprouted, their vitamin content sometimes increases hundreds of times. This is also another indication of Yin.

"C is the vitamin we should worry about most because not only is it unstable ($\triangledown$), but it cannot be stored in the body and it drains away rapidly under conditions of cold, heat, fatigue, and stress; this last being a condition from which millions more suffer today that at any time in the past." (See P.E. Norris' excellent book, *About Vitamins.*)

Furthermore, cooking and pressure-cooking destroy much of the Vitamin C in all foods. This is the reason many health-minded people are against the Macrobiotic diet.

This is not a just claim, however; cooking or not cooking makes little difference because the strong acid and alkaline in the body, as well as the body temperature, destroy the Vitamin C anyway, as Mr. Henaff points out. The average man must be able to produce his own Vitamin C as does the Eskimo. Japanese scientists claim that tea leaves contain pro-vitamin C which turns to Vitamin C after heating. Scurvy has never been widespread in Japan even though the Japanese eat almost all cooked foods. Dr. McCollum, professor of Biochemistry at John Hopkins University said in his book, *The Newer Knowledge of Nutrition*, that animals are able to produce Vitamin C by themselves. Why isn't man able to produce it any more? Is this a sign of degeneration? Animal experiments show that mice fed foods lacking in Vitamin C over a long period of time, sustain their life without suffering from scurvy. This is the result of Vitamin C production by the mice themselves (Parson, 1920). According to McCollum, only the human being, marmot, and monkey are not able to produce Vitamin C. Mice, dogs, pigeons, chickens, duck, turkeys and pheasants do not need Vitamin C at all. Could the inability of man and monkey to produce Vitamin C be a result of eating too much Vitamin C, such as that found in fruits? According to Mr. Ohsawa, man will be able to produce his own Vitamin C if he stops eating a large amount of fruits. One who is afraid of a Vitamin C shortage in his diet, can eat salted, pressed salad or raw salad - (without salt). (Pressed salad after every meal is very satisfying.)

2. Vitamin A.

According to the modern nutrition theories, animals can not produce the A vitamins. Vegetables also cannot synthesize it. Therefore, scientists believe that carotene, which plants synthesize, turns to Vitamin A in the animal body.

Exposure to heat and air tends to destroy Vitamin A and carotene, but if there is heat only and no air, the vitamin is not affected. This indicates that Vitamin A is more yang than Vitamin C. Because there is so much Vitamin A in so many foods, and excess Vitamin A can be stored in the liver, the risk of a deficiency is small in the Macrobiotic diet, even on Regimen #7, if Miso soup is eaten daily.

3. Vitamin B_1 (known as Thiamine)

This is one of the most important vitamins. A serious shortage of B_1 can cause the following: 1) loss of appetite 2) indigestion, alternating with constipation and possible colitis (inflamation of the colon or large bowel) 3) inflammation of the heart and heart trouble 4) numbness or pain in the fingers or arms.

P.E. Norris states in *About Vitamins* that, "B_1 is partly destroyed in the body and passed out in the urine, and the body will not store it. Therefore, it must be constantly replenished."

According to Dr. McCollum, B_1 is not destroyed by normal cooking if the pH is less than 7 (an acid condition). Macrobiotic cooking, especially pressure-cooking, will destroy B_1. The situation, however, is similar to that of Vitamin

C; destroying B_1 by cooking doesn't change the value of the food much, because B_1 will be destroyed by digestion due to the alkaline condition in the intestines. Therefore, we must produce our own B_1. Vitamin B_1 contained in foods may help in this production after its decomposition. If we eat whole grains which are rich in B_1, we will get B_1 even though it is destroyed by cooking. Since refined starches lack B_1 those foods such as white sugar, refined flour and polished rice should be avoided.

Another interesting fact about B_1 is that it can be produced from the cellulose of vegetable foods in the large intestine, with the help of bacteria. Macrobiotic teaching recommends eating whole foods which contain cellulose. Even this so-called waste can be a very important source of the B vitamin. Here we see the wonderful mechanism and constitution of Nature. Nature gives us everything. If we eat whole foods, we will have whole nourishment. Thus, we don't need any supplements. We don't need to worry about the latest findings or new drugs, if we live on the Macrobiotic diet which guarantees us a healthy stomach and strong intestines.

4. Vitamin B_2 (Riboflavin)

According to P.E. Norris, the shortage of B_2 causes reddening of facial skin and cracking at the edges of the mouth. Also, the corners of the eyes and insides of the eyelids grow sore. In India, millions of people who live on food deficient in B_2 (white rice, for instance) develop cataracts. B_2 is found abundantly in yeast, fresh raw milk, leafy green vegetables such as turnips and carrot tops, broccoli, spinach, lettuce, cabbage, and the germ and bran of wheat and bran of rice. Therefore, in the Macrobiotic diet, there will be no deficiency of B_2.

From the standpoint of Macrobiotics, cracks at the edge of the mouth are a sign of a bad stomach (over-eating) and sores on the eyelid are a sign of kidney trouble. Therefore, I suspect that B_2 must be related to the function of the stomach and kidney.

5. Vitamin B_{12}.

B_{12} is a recent addition to the list of vitamins. A shortage of B_{12} according to modern nutrition causes "pernicious anemics" which are now treated with injections of from 10 to 100 micrograms of B_{12}. Not only does B_{12} restore the constituents of the blood to normal, it improves the general well-being of the sick. Liver seems to be rich in B_{12}. (The Chinese medicine for anemia is an extract from cow's liver, which must contain B_{12}.) According to modern science, B is a vitamin containing cobalt which enables us to convert iron into red blood cells. According to Macrobiotic teaching, B_{12} is an enzyme or intermediate substance which can promote chemical reactions and the transmutation of elements.

Dr. K. Morishita claims that we are able to manufacture B_{12} from cellulose in the large intestine as we do in the case of B_1 and B_6. We recommend that anemic persons eat whole small fish. In severe cases of anemia, pheasant meat or fowl liver is recommended. According to the Macrobiotic principle, the plasma is formed by the intestines and then is transmuted to red and white cells. Therefore, healthy intestines and chewing well are the most important aspects in curing anemia. One who observes the Macrobiotic diet for awhile will not find it necessary to take B_{12} pills. Pregnant women who tend to be anemic should eat Miso soup and small fish regularly. (Beginners of Macrobiotics may eat fowl.) If they are not able to eat Miso soup - if they are too yang - they should eat Miso spread (a mixture of Miso and Tahini), scallion Miso, white fish meat, mochi, or sometimes eggs. (Note: too much egg is bad for the eyes and liver.)

Look at the following lists carefully. Cabbage, carrots, broccoli, Chinese cabbage, cauliflower, corn, lettuce, and squash are rich in all vitamins. For that reason, the Macrobiotic diet which recommends those vegetables provides the sufficient amount of vitamins. Any vitamin deficiency is due to the inability to assimilate them because of bad intestines. One who has bad intestines should chew well - more than 100 times. Since Vitamin C is very yin, a yin person should avoid foods with high Vitamin C content.

Yang persons should choose foods rich in Vitamin C. Horseradish and daikon (white Japanese radish) contain a large amount of Vitamin C; they are always used with fish which is yang. Use these tables as a guide of Yin and Yang in cooking, preparing the menu, and serving.

Tables are not necessary if you understand the Macrobiotic Yin-Yang principle. You can select food by Yin and Yang, which actually allows for a better selection of foods, because these tables are an indication of average and not individual foods. The food value changes with climate, locality, soil condition, fertilizer, way of storing, period of storing, etc.

Vitamin contents in 1 lb. of various foods: (From Composition of Foods, U.S. Government Dept. of Agriculture)

	Vit. A(I.U.)	Vit. B_1 (mg)	Vit. B_2 (mg)	Niacine (mg)	Vit. C (mg)
Abalone	-	.54	-	-	-
Almond	0	.22	4.20	15.9	0
Apple	380	.12	.08	.3	16
Bacon	0	1.64	.52	8.3	-
Barley	0	.55	.23	14.1	0
Lima Beans	530	.43	.22	2.5	52
Mung beans	360	1.71	.96	11.7	-
Beef	320	.23	.47	12.8	-
Beer	-	.01	.13	2.9	-
Blackberry	860	.14	.18	1.6	90
Wholewheat Bread	-	1.17	.56	12.9	-
Broccoli	8,840	.35	.81	3.2	400
Buckwheat	0	2.71	-	20	0
Butter	15,000	-	-	-	0
Cabbage	530	.22	.20	1.3	192
Chinese Cabbage	660	.20	.18	2.5	110
Carp	230	.01	.05	2	2
Carrot	29,440	.16	.14	1.6	21
Cauliflower	270	.50	.44	3	354
Celery	820	.09	.11	1.2	30
Cheese	5,940	.12	2.07	.3	0
Chicken	1,600	.14	.82	12.1	-
Corn	650	.24	.19	2.8	20
Egg	4,760	.42	1.20	.2	0

	Vit. A	Vit. B_1	Vit. B_2	Niacine	Vit. C
Grapes	290	.15	.08	.7	10
Honey	0	.02	.2	1.2	5
Horseradish	-	.23	-	-	268
Lettuce	3,260	.21	.2	.9	28
Lime	50	.10	.08	.7	141
Lamb liver	229,070	1.81	14.89	76.5	152
Milk	650	.15	.78	.3	5
Onion	160	.14	.15	.8	42
Orange	620	.3	.12	1.2	188
Peanuts (roasted)	-	1.45	.60	77.8	0
Pork	0	1.58	.36	8.5	-
Potato	-	.39	.14	5.4	73
Pumpkin	5,080	.14	.35	1.8	30
Raisin	100	.51	.37	2.4	5
Radish	40	.13	.12	1.3	106
Daikon	40	.11	.07	1.3	113
Brown Rice	0	1.52	.24	21.4	0
Rice Bran	0	10.25	1.14	135.4	0
Sesame seeds	140	4.43	1.08	24.3	0
Soybeans	3,130	2	.72	6.2	130
Spinach	36,740	.44	.91	2.8	231
Squash	1,800	.23	.38	4.5	95
Strawberry	260	.12	.29	2.6	257
Wheat	0	2.59	.54	19.5	0
Brewer's yeast	-	70.81	19.41	171.9	-

These tables are for beginners who are not able to select foods by the Yin-Yang principle. You can discard these when you learn Yin and Yang. In this list of the vitamins found in various foods, lamb liver has the highest content of all vitamins. Actually, any animal liver contains a similar amount of vitamins. Why? Isn't it strange? Vitamins are not stable in heat and alkaline conditions, as are found in the liver. How can the liver store such high amount of vitamins? Is this not an indication that the yang liver constantly manufactures yin vitamins?

H. CONCLUSION - 8 Macrobiotic Principles

What is Macrobiotics? There are as many ideas about this as there are people who have ever heard the word. But here, as I see it, are the 8 most basic Macrobiotic principles:

1. Ecology

In the primarily carnivorous Western world, this word is a new one. Ecology, in the West, would probably not have gained its present popularity if it were not for Western man's fear of pollution and "over-population". This fear is one side of a coin whose other side is the conquer nature mentality. In the primarily herbiverous East, where one has tended to aim for co-operation with nature, the word "ecology" is at least 4,000 years old. In China, it was expressed by the following 4 words: Shin (body) Do (soil) Fu (not) Ji (two): Body and soil are not two; they are one. The soil produces plants, which are eaten by animals and used by them to make their blood, cells, tissues and organs. Man, an animal, is a transmutation of the soil. In *Man, the Unknown*, Alexis Carrel says, "Man is literally made from the dust of the earth. For this reason, his physiological and mental activities are profoundly influenced by the geological constitution of the country where he lives, by the nature of the animals and plants that he eats."

Man is healthy and strong when he lives on the products of his nearby surroundings, ideally by growing his own food. Man, the freest animal, can adjust to almost any climate. But we must keep certain factors (temperature, water, sugar and mineral levels, etc.) quite constant, merely to stay alive, and even more constant if we want to be healthy. And the best foods for maintaining constancy of physiological and mental conditions are those that are locally grown.

2. Economy of Life

Modern man, who considers money essential to his happiness emphasizes economy of money, with the result that many people save their money and lose their lives. Money does bring us some happiness, by helping us to satisfy certain basic needs. But when we are unsatisfied with such satisfactions and greedily seek more and more comfort, convenience and luxury, we are contributing to the loss of our happiness.

For the past 40-50 years, for example, most of our farmers have been basing their practices on economy of money - by using insecticides and fertilizers in order to produce larger yields, and thus greater profits, to satisfy their greed; this is not economy of life. The insecticides kill many organisms that are essential to a healthy soil (and thus also to healthy plants and animals which are the products of that soil); and the fertilizers acidify and otherwise weaken the soil, also. Too much emphasis on short-run big yields for higher profits is breaking the patterns of natural life, which is self-destructive. Also, such unnatural practices, sooner or later, weaken the soil so much that even profits diminish. So in the long run, economy of life turns out to be economy of money too but not vice versa. Crop rotation and the use of organic fertilizers (returning to the soil what we cannot use for food) are enough to assure us of a continuous supply of food that will keep us strong.

Economy of life is applied in our diet as "no waste". (It is not at all uncommon for a Zen monk to be severely scolded for leaving a single grain of rice on the kitchen floor.) The less food we waste, the more there is for others - one of the most obvious solutions to the "over-population problem". The amount of food thrown away in stores, restaurants and homes all over America is astounding.

In terms of the foods we eat, economy of life is observed in our trying to eat mainly whole foods. When we eat only parts of foods, we become malnourished, and our metabolism becomes unbalanced. When you eat fish, for example, do you eat the whole thing - tail, bones, head, and all the rest? If not - if you eat only the flesh (rich in protein and fat) - your blood will become acid, whereas if you also eat the other parts (rich in minerals, including calcium, magnesium, iodine and many others), your body will be able to neutralize the acidity more easily. One reason carnivorous animals are able to maintain balanced body conditions is that they eat whole foods. (Another is their great amount of activity, which helps them transmute what they eat into what their bodies need.)

Because they are not whole foods, refined sugar and all other synthetic chemicals are not conducive to our health. They are "pure", which is why they are harmful. When we eat grain-, vegetable-, bean-, fruit-, and nut-sugars (or even the sugar of organically grown, unprocessed honey), we are also taking into our bodies many vitamins and minerals that we need to digest them.

The same applies to all examples of discarding part of a whole food, such as wheat germ, vitamin pills, white flour and refined salt. Let us look at refined salt as a typical example: It is almost nothing but sodium and chlorine (unless it has been "fortified" with synthetic iodine - "iodized"), whereas "crude" salt is rich in many other minerals (including iodine).

These first two principles - ecology and economy of life - may be summed up as natural eating and farming: to nourish oneself primarily with untreated, locally grown whole foods, and to return to the soil those of its products which we cannot use as food, and thus keep ourselves and our soil (which are one) healthy and whole.

3. The Yin-Yang Principle

This is our guiding compass. It shows us our direction in life in much the same way a North-South compass shows us geographical direction. The Yin-Yang ("unifying") principle is a useful tool for us. It can help us find our position in the infinite universe and it can also lead us to health and happiness by enabling us to analyze the foods we eat and their effects on our bodies and minds.

Anything at all can be analyzed in terms of Yin and Yang - which is really just another way of saying that everything in this constantly changing world is relative. For example, think of color. This whole universe is a magnetic field of positive and negative charges which is constantly vibrating and thus producing electro-magnetic waves. Some of these waves are then perceived by our nervous system and translated by our brain into what we call "the spectrum of colors":

untraviolet-violet-indigo-blue-green-yellow-brown-orange-red-infrared
- visible -

Red gives us a feeling of warmth and excitement (movement); so we call it "Yang". We see centrifugality (expansiveness) and centripetality (contractiveness) as the 2 forces that are the first manifestations of the relative world, and which produce all others. We call then "Yin" and "Yang" respectively - though any other two words expressing oppositeness (contrast) would do just as well. By observation, logic and intuition, we then place the following in the Yang category: time, movement, inside, male, animal, etc.; and the following in the Yin category: space, rest, outside, female, plant, etc. Violet gives us a feeling of coolness and serenity (rest), so we call it Yin. But Yin and Yang are relative terms always; so blue, for example, is yin compared to green, and yang compared to violet. The plant world is represented by green (from our perception of chlorophyll) and the animal world by red (the color of hemoglobin). Man's physiological spectrum normally runs from red to yellow. Man is a yang animal; and that is one reason we are so strongly attracted to yin foods - especially when we are eating a lot of yang foods - because Yang attracts Yin (and Yin attracts Yang).

The following table is a rough approximation of the Yin-Yang spectrum of foods and a corresponding table of colors as a means of discussing those foods. This table is not cut and dried, and there are some exceptions; some foods in a more yin category are more yang than others in a more yang one. For example, burdock is a land vegetable, a more yin category than beans; but soybeans are more yin than burdock, because soybeans are a very yin bean, and burdock is a very yang land vegetable.

∇ (Yin) - synthetic drugs - natural drugs - sugar - oil - yeast - honey - fruit - water - nuts - sea vegetables - land vegetables - beans - grains - shellfish - miso - fish - soy sauce - crude salt - fowl - meat - eggs - refined salt - △ (Yang)

∇ (Yin) - ultraviolet - violet - indigo - blue - green - yellow -

brown - orange - red - infrared - △ (Yang)

(Dairy products are very difficult to place in such a classification, since some (goat milk, goat cheese, roquefort, edam) are very △ (about as yang as miso) and others (cream, yogurt) are very ▽ (about as ▽ as honey). Cow's milk and most cheeses and butters are in between. As for alcoholic beverages, most are very ▽ (between oil and sugar) but some (naturally fermented sake, beer) are only about as ▽ as fruit. Alcohol, by the way, has a faster effect than sugar, but its effects go away in 1-2 days in most cases, whereas sugar's effects are generally felt for at least a week - not to mention these effects which are not so noticeable and last longer.

Although I have suggested that man's physiological spectrum normally runs from yellow to red, we can maintain balanced conditions even if we eat some "green" foods (fruits through green land vegetables or even some "blue" ones (oil, yeast, honey) if we don't eat them often or in large quantities. And, by the same token, anything more △ than crude salt, though generally not harmful if taken only very occasionally, depending on the individual and many constantly changing environmental factors, is not conducive to our health as daily food in this climatic zone. Naturally, anything more yin than oil in the above table should be very strongly avoided - especially synthetic drugs.

It is interesting that the above suggestions, based on the ▽/△ principle, fit very nicely with the first 2 (ecology and economy of life.) Even what might appear to be an exception (natural drugs) is really not because in our climatic zone there are very few natural drugs. Most that are used are either synthetic, imported, or have been transplanted from more tropical areas. Importing is against ecology (local foods) and transplanting is really the same thing; it is very unnatural to force a plant to change its eating habits so fast. It generally takes a couple of hundred years before a plant from a tropical zone can adapt to a temperate one - if it does manage to do so. This is one reason that the drugs which have been transplanted here are so much weaker than those which are imported directly from the country of origin.

In terms of our mentality, ▽ foods tend to cause ▽ emotions and thinking (fear, suspicion, deceit, etc.),△ foods, △ emotions and thinking (hostility, noisiness, brusqueness, etc.) and a good balance (✡) tends to lead us to harmony and peace.

How do we maintain a balanced pattern of eating?

In all but extremely cold (▽) climates - where our main foods are meat and fish (△) - grains and vegetables are our main foods, as they are nearest the balance of a healthy human being. If we eat fish in a warmer climate, we need a lot of raw vegetables or even fruit (▽) to balance it. Except in extremely cold climates, we avoid meat, as it is so △ we would need large amounts of fruit or honey to balance it, and we try to avoid eating large amounts of foods that are not in the middle line of the previous table. Sugar is so extremely ▽ that it is impossible to balance it; but honey, if organically grown and unprocessed, can be used once in a while by most people without harm - especially in warm weather. (One teaspoon of such honey is less ▽ than 5 or 6 apples. Quantity, it is helpful to remember, changes quality. A big amount, relative to a small one, is ▽ .)

In tropical areas or summer in temperate ones, we need less salt, fish, grains, and more water, nuts, fruits. (Is it not clear by now that to speak of "the Macrobiotic diet" as a set thing is false?)

If we want to analyze foods as ▽ or △ , we need to consider many factors, such as climate of origin (hot (△) climates produce ▽ foods; they, and we, become more ▽ as a way of adapting); direction and location of growth (up, above ground are ▽); speed of growth (fast is ▽); density (greater is △); shape (round, compact, small are △); chemical composition (sodium, carbon, hydrogen are △ ; most others are ▽); and so on.

Time, heat, pressure and salt are yangizing; they all shift the color spectrum of foods towards the red side. By using them, we can eat some fairly ▽ foods and still maintain good balance. And by using less △ factors and more ▽ ones (spices, water, fruit, etc.), we can eat some fairly △ foods, too. Macrobiotic cooking is a technique which enables us to enjoy both the taste and appearance of our foods and their effects on our bodies and minds.

Good balance of ▽ and △ is our goal and our guide. Since most of us are unbalanced on the ▽ side (though we may also be too △ in some ways) we are trying to become more △ ; but to do so, we must sometimes take ▽ detours: "Five steps backward; six steps forward!" "Limitation, success. Galling limitation must not be persevered in." (I CHING). Following very broad guidelines leads to success. Carefully analyzing each mouthful of food or limiting one's eating pattern too strictly turns to its opposite (chaos - "bingeing" - loss of balance). If you have been eating meat and sugar, or (especially) taking drugs in the past 5 years or so, then simply by eating mainly locally grown whole foods from oil to crude salt in the above table, your health will improve greatly. And you will have plenty of room in which to enjoy a relaxed and quite variable diet - which is not only conducive to your maintaining a balanced pattern of eating; it will also allow your body and mind to adjust gradually to the changes they will be going through.

4. Transmutation
Macrobiotics differs from any other Western diets or nutrition theories because it is based on the transmutation theory. The philosphy of transmutation has been taught in the East for thousands of years. I CHING is nothing but the teaching of transmutation - change. The Haramitta Sutra teaches that all phenomena are transmuted manifestations of Oneness.

The Biological Atomic Transmutation theory was coined by Mr. L. Kervran and Mr. George Ohsawa. Mr. Ohsawa said in his condensation of *Biological Transmutation,* "After thirteen years of experiment and observation, Kervran and Prof. Baranger (the latter is of the Polytechnology School in Paris) reached the wonderful conclusion that elements transmute to other elements in the biological body." Na becomes K. K changes to Ca. Na changes to Mg. Na becomes

CO, etc. All these phenomenal changes occur in the biological body.

For 2,000 years the atom was considered the basic fundamental unit of stable elements, but it isn't any more. The atom also changes.

The atomic conception in physiology is "all cells come only from cells," created by Virchow, the German physicist. This belief in the constancy of the cell is the basic concept of modern biology, physiology, and medicine. Therefore, such a concept eliminates a connection between foods, cells, organs, body and mind. This is the most important short coming of modern medicine.

According to Dr. K. Morishita, "Modern medicine and biology teach that cells grow by the division of cells. For example, one liver cell will divide into two, two into four, etc. This is true only under special conditions, like in a vitro (test tube). It never happens, however, in the normal living body."

"From my study the red cells gather and form the various organs and tissues. Therefore, our body is a transformation of food. Our constitution and character depend upon our food. Food is life. In conclusion, in our body the digested food (which is organic matter) transforms itself into the simplest life (a red cell); and this simple life is transformed to a higher stage of life - a body cell. According to my theory of evolution, there once existed only inorganic matter on the earth. Then the inorganic changed to organic matter, the organic matter to protein and the protein to simple life. The coordination of this simple life developed to the higher life of animals and then finally reached the stage of man. This fantastic evolution of life is not a mere theory of anthropology. It is taking place in our body every day, every second. It has taken billions of years to evolve from the inorganic stage to man. In our body it takes only one or two days. What a miracle we have been doing." (See *The Hidden Truth of Cancer.*)

Without the concept of transmutation, animal life is separate from plant life, plant life has no connection with soil or water, and soil and water have no relation to solar energy.

Everything is part of a totality but there is no unification. The result is confusion and symptomatic medicine which is based on an anatomical concept of life.

Our body is under constant change - foods have to be digested to amino acids, fat, or glucose. Glucose is converted to glycogen, which in turn changes back to glucose when the sugar level goes down. Organic matter changes to body cells. The end of these changes is to maintain certain constancies - constancy in body temperature, acidity or alkalinity, concentration of elements, sugar level, amount of O_2, amount of CO_2, amount of body fluid, and amount of blood.

Change or transmutation makes a state of constancy in our body condition possible. Without transmutation, there is no universal constancy. Without constancy, there is no life. Constancy and transmutation are two sides - the front and back - of life. Medicine and nutrition are like a snap-shot picture. They overlook the fact of transmutation. Their theory cannot explain life. The modern nutrition theory is inadequate to explain why Eskimoes have the most Vitamin C in their blood compared to other people, when they eat the least amount of fresh vegetables. (See *Vitamin C and Fruits* - Macroguide #6). The modern physiologist who believes in blood formation in bone marrow cannot explain the fact that soldiers who lost arms or legs can maintain the normal blood amount. (Arms and legs constitute a large portion of the bone marrow in our body.)

Biology cannot explain the following fact:

"Chickens feeding on a clay soil were left without limestone. When the eggs appeared to have a soft shell, mica was given. The very next day hard shells reappeared! (Keep in mind that while the interior of the egg reflects the food taken weeks before, its shell does not show a trace of an element taken more than forty-eight hours before.) Similar experiments were conducted with guinea hens which had been laying eggs with hard shells every other day. Mica was fed and the shells produced were hard every day. The experiment continued for forty-three days during which time the supply of mica was interrupted on several occasions. The day after the mica was withheld, a soft-shelled egg appeared.

67

Mica was restored to the diet: a hard egg reappeared the day afterward." (*Biological Transmutation*, by L. Kervran - Book condensation by George Ohsawa)

How does the concept of transmutation apply to the diet? First, eat foods which strengthen transmutation ability, such as vegetal food, including grains, vegetables, beans, and seaweed. Second, cooking destroys vitamins and enzymes. However, it yangizes food. Therefore, we improve the ability of transmutation. As a result, we can produce our own vitamins and enzymes. Third, eat less foods which have a high vitamin content. This is contrary to the modern nutrition theory.

Note: Persons whose diet included a high intake of milk, meat or fruit and drugs lost their ability of transmutation and must change to this diet gradually.

5. An Art of Living

Macrobiotics is not a science whose goal is the accumulation of knowledge. Knowledge has meaning only when it can lead us to health and happiness.

Modern science analyzes, and then brings forth theories and "laws", all of which are attempts to find absolute truth in the relative world, and which, moreover, have little if anything to do with health and, more importantly, happiness.

Macrobiotics, on the other hand, is an art. Knowing that no absolute rules exist, or can be followed forever, we start with principles that are as adaptable to the constantly changing world we inhabit as possible. Only you are the artist who draws the painting of your life. Macrobiotics is neither rigidity nor imitation.

General directions are perhaps necessary for most people when they begin following a Macrobiotic way of life. But as you experiment, observe yourself, and learn the Yin-Yang principle, you will gain the ability to make your life as interesting, exciting and amusing as you wish.

We humans are passengers on an express train called Earth - a short, limited trip. Let's enjoy this trip and amuse ourselves as much as possible! Macrobiotics is the art of doing so.

In school, we are taught to memorize facts and information. Our judgment then is based mainly on this collected data which has many limitations. When it comes to everyday life, this memorized information is inadequate or confusing in its ability to lead us to a happier life. Only our higher and better judgment which is developed from our daily experiences can lead us to solve our daily problems. For example, we give people advice concerning what and how much to eat or drink. However, this advice should be varied depending on an individual's consititution, his daily activities, the climate in which he is living, etc.

Strictly speaking, no one eats the same food and same amount even from the same cooking pot. Such recognition of individuality leads us to the fact that we are living by ourselves and we are creating our life by ourselves. During the fetal period, we created our heart, brain, stomach, kidney, liver, arms, legs and other parts of our body. After we were born, we improved our body function through talking, walking, perceiving, feeling, thinking, etc. However, this development of self often ceases when school education forces us to memorize facts and information instead of learning methods of improving our judgment. As the result, modern people cannot judge what to eat and drink or how much to eat and drink. Because they live on the judgment of others, these individuals are not living by themselves. Their lives are not their own anymore. Therefore, during periods of sickness or difficulties, they do not know what to do and fall into periods of deep depression and lose their minds.

If one lives and depends upon himself at all times, he can find the way to overcome any difficulties. Macrobiotics teaches such a way of life through an artistic living because macrobiotics creates beauty in body and mind.

In modern society, artists are special and gifted people. However, the macrobiotic way of living turns everyone into an artist because one begins creating by himself a life directed towards greater beauty and health.

Macrobiotics is an art of living that is joyful, amusing, happy, healthy, and free. It is based on the realization that only you are the master of yourself - not bacteria, doctors,

69

scientists, ministers, philosophers or dieticians - especially not Macrobiotic ones!

6. Appreciation

Macrobiotics is neither merely a way of curing illness nor a mystical Oriental cuisine. Some people think it's a brown rice diet, others that it means giving up pleasure at meals. How far from the truth all these ideas are! Macrobiotics is a profound understanding of the orderliness of nature, a practical application of which enables us to prepare attractive, delicious meals and achieve a happy and free life. The 6th and most important principle of Macrobiotics is appreciation (gratitude). Why? Because it is the cause of freedom and happiness. Without it, there can be no freedom and happiness.

There are many rich people who commit suicide. Eastman and Nobel were unhappy despite their fortunes. Why? Because they did not appreciate their wealth. There are, on the other hand, many people who would be so happy to be given $5.00 that they would never forget it and would give back appreciation to the giver.

Most of us lack gratitude. We tend to remember what we have given, and forget what we have been given. Living this way, we complain, and live an unhappy, unsatisfied, unfree life. We forget that we have been given everything we need - air, light, water and food - freely and with no strings attached, since birth. We forget the infinite generosity and tolerance of our mother Infinity, who lets us live and play even when we don't show her any gratitude.

Macrobiotics is an attempt to experience and express gratitude towards everything, beginning with a grain of rice, a bowl of soup or a piece of bread. It teaches us to appreciate everything without exception, including pain, disease, hatred, and intolerance. How can we appreciate such things? By realizing that they are our teachers, which help us to see our ignorance, prejudice, intolerance, and exclusiveness. When we appreciate such things, we manifest the highest judgment - the objectivity of the infinite universe, which appreciates everything, including our intolerant selves.

Macrobiotic eating gives us a bodily condition which helps us express gratitude. But if you do not appreciate your life, then you might as well get sick, and appreciate your sickness. There are many people who are healthy but unhappy, and there are others who are sick and happy. Why is this?

> "All animals and vegetables return thousands of times more than they receive. One grain is given to the earth; the earth gives back several thousand . . . Some female fish give billions of eggs. Such is the natural biological law. Your parents have given you life - take care of them infinitely. When they are gone, help the parents of others, indirectly or directly. This is the Oriental concept of ON, which is much more than the discharging of a debt. ON is joyfulness in distributing eternal happiness and infinite freedom." *(Zen Macrobiotics)*

7. Faith

Our red blood cells change completely every 3 months. When we begin eating Macrobiotically, our red blood cells thus become healthier very quickly. The fantastic improvements most people experience in the first three months of such eating are fairly easily achieved. But the improvements which take place after 3 months are more gradual and difficult. One may even experience an occasional worsening of one's condition.

Why does this happen? The main reason is as follows: After the change in red blood cells comes a change in intercellular fluid (between cells). Nutritive substances from the intercellular fluid entering the body cells begin gradually making them healthier. Like everything else, however, body cells are characterized by a front and a back (2 sides of the same coin; either could be called front or back, depending on one's point of view), one of which is the tendency to remain constant and the other is the ability to adapt. The body cells of most people beginning Macrobiotic eating are weak in adapting; they are too constant (rigid) - as opposed to the red blood cells and intercellular fluid, which change more easily because they are not so "established". So the body cells resist (do not easily adapt to) the new intercellular fluid. It is this resistance to change by the body cells which is usually the cause of temporary worsenings of conditions in people who have been eating Macrobiotically for about 4 months to a year. It is the same kind of resistance we see in the struggle between the older, more established conservatives and the younger, more flexible radicals.

When such a worsening of conditions occurs, many people tend to feel that it is because Macrobiotics is not the right way of eating. At such times, a clear understanding of Macrobiotics is important.

True faith is not a superficial belief (credo) or superstition. It is clear understanding of Oneness (the entire infinite universe and all of its infinite manifestations); we are manifestions of Oneness. We are the center of a spiral that begins in The Void and passes through Yin and Yang, energy, sub-atomic particles, elements, plants and animals - each stage being a transmutation of the stage which precedes it. This spiral is a continuity. Light, air, water and food are around us in abundance. (Pollution can be described as over-population control by the order of the universe - justice). Light, air, water, grains, land vegetables, sea vegetables, beans, nuts, fish, fruit, salt and animal foods are available to us, in that approximate order; and that is the approximate order in which we must eat them if we want to be healthy. Since Macrobiotics shows us a sensible order of foods, it is sensible to eat Macrobiotically. If my condition worsens, it is due to: (a) expelling of toxins and/or excess, (b) body cell resistance to new intercellular fluid, and/or (c) the inaccurate application of Macrobiotics.

Without such faith, you may wander from one way of eating to another, in vain, and become extremely confused. But with such faith (common sense), you will not become confused or disturbed by any temporary worsening of conditions.

However, faith in Macrobiotics must be clearly distinguished from stubborness or rigidity. If a person's condition worsens continuously, he would be wise to consider the possibility that his application of Macrobiotics is inaccurate, and to consult with someone whose judgment is clearer or has had more Macrobiotic experience. He may not be eating broadly enough.

"Faith is not a creed, but a clear-sighted understanding of the order of the universe, through all the finite, transient and illusory phenomena, internally; and, externally, of the Love that embraces everything without exclusiveness . . . the biggest thing in life is faith." *(The Book of Judgment)*

"Since nature has provided us with foods that are proper for our bodies, we can achieve health by recognizing and using them. This is Macrobiotics, the materialization of the order of nature in our eating and drinking. If we live with awareness to this order, health can result. If we do not, disease is more likely to follow. This is simple, clear and practical. It is justice." *(Zen Macrobiotics)*

8. Do-o-Raku

Do-o is the Japanese equivalent of the Chinese word Tao, the order of nature. Raku means "enjoyment". To enjoy Tao (to live with appreciation all the time, wherever we are) is Do-o-Raku. When we are aware of nature's impartial and absolute justice, we know there is nothing to worry about. In Lin Chi's words: "At one stroke I forgot all my knowledge! There's no need for any discipline; for, move as I will, I always manifest the Tao!" When we see this, we can begin to enjoy our lives fully, by distributing infinite joy and thankfulness to everyone we meet.

Interestingly, Do-o-Raku also means "hobby". So we can say that Do-o-Raku means to live our life as a hobby - which is what it is! Anything we do is a game. It does not matter if we "fail" or "succeed". Such an understanding is Nirvana - eternal peace. In the words of Paramahansa Yogananda: "Do not take life's experiences too seriously . . . for in reality they are nothing but dream experiences. Play your part in life, but never forget that it is only a role.

To live in perpetual ecstatic delight is Do-o-Raku. Those who do so are called Do-o-Raku-Mono. If you are Do-o-Raku-Mono, you are Macrobiotic, whatever you eat.

The Unifying Principle: 12 Dynamic Theorems Which Describe the Creation and Functioning of the Relative World:

1. Oneness (infinite expansion) continuously manifests itself, at all points and moments, as divisions of itself which create 2 forces: centrifugality (expansiveness) and centripetality (contractiveness).

2. Let us call centrifugality "Yin", and centripetality "Yang".

3. Yin and Yang are constantly changing into each other.

4. At the extremes of development, Yin produces or becomes Yang and Yang produces or becomes Yin.

5. Yin attracts Yang and Yang attracts Yin.

6. The force of attraction between Yin and Yang is greater when the difference between them is greater, and smaller when it is smaller.

7. Yin repels Yin and Yang repels Yang.

8. The force of repulsion between Yin and Yang is smaller when the difference between them is greater, and greater when it is smaller.

9. Yin and Yang, combined in an infinite variety of proportions, produce energy and all other phenomena, visible and invisible.

10. No phenomenon is only yin or only yang; all phenomena are composed of both Yin and Yang.

11. No phenomenon is balanced; all phenomena are composed of unequal proportions of Yin and Yang.

12. All phenomena are yang at the center and yin at the surface.

The Order of the Universe: 7 Dynamic Universal Principles Which Describe the Relative World and Its Relationship to Oneness:

1. All visible and invisible phenomena are manifestations of Oneness.

2. All visible and invisible phenomena are different from all others.

3. All visible and invisible phenomena are constantly changing.

4. All visible and invisible phenomena have a beginning and an end.

5. All visible and invisible phenomena have a front and a back.

6. The bigger the front, the bigger the back.

7. All antagonisms are complimentary.

These principles above are all dynamic (dialectical) - as opposed to formal (Aristotelian) logic, which is as static and rigid as a snap-shot and can never represent real Life.